Successful
Breastfeeding

D0485031

This handbook is dedicated with respect and affection to Dr Mavis Gunther. The members of the group have had to re-learn much of what Dr Gunther already knew in the 1940s, 50s and 60s; at last, in the 1980s, we are able to write a handbook of breastfeeding which has been inspired by her sound clinical understanding and her rigorous scientific approach.

For Churchill Livingstone:

Publisher: Mary Law
Editorial co-ordination: Editorial Resources Unit
Production controller: Nancy Henry
Design: Design Resources Unit
Sales Promotion Executive: Hilary Brown

Successful Breastfeeding

Royal College of Midwives

Second edition

ROYAL COLLEGE
OF MIDWIVES
LONDON 1991

CHURCHILL LIVINGSTONE
EDINBURGH LONDON MELBOURNE
NEW YORK AND TOKYO 1991

CHURCHILL LIVINGSTONE
Medical Division of Longman Group UK Limited

Distributed in the United States of America by Churchill Livingstone
Inc., 1560 Broadway, New York, N.Y. 10036, and by associated
companies, branches and representatives throughout the world.

Royal College of Midwives
15 Mansfield Street
London W1M OBE
Tel. 071–580 6523

First edition (Royal College of Midwives) 1988
Second edition (Churchill Livingstone) 1991

ISBN 0-443-04460-0

British Library Cataloguing in Publication Data
Successful breastfeeding.
1. Babies. Breast feeding
I. Royal College of Midwives
649.33

Library of Congress Cataloging in Publication Data
Successful breastfeeding/Royal College of Midwives. – 1st CL ed.
p.   cm.
Includes bibliographical references.
Includes index.
ISBN 0-443-04460-0
1. Breast feeding.   I. Royal College of Midwives (Great Britain)
[DNLM: 1. Breastfeeding.   WS 125 S942]
RJ216.S874   1991
649'.33 – dc20
DNLM/DLC   90–15049
for Library of Congress   CIP

Illustrations: Joanne Moon
                Mike Woolridge (Fig. 15)
Produced by Longman Singapore Publishers Pte Ltd
Printed in Singapore

Preface

A breastfeeding working group was set up by the Council
of the Royal College of Midwives in May 1986, in
response to a challenge issued by the December 1985
meeting of the Royal Society of Medicine's Forum on
Maternity and the Newborn. The subject of that meeting
was 'Difficulties with Breastfeeding – Midwives in
Disarray?' (1). There it was acknowledged that for a
variety of reasons there was very little consistency
between breastfeeding policies in different parts of the
country and also between policy and practice within many
individual institutions. Furthermore, it was apparent that
many current practices (and policies) were not only
unsupported by research evidence but in some cases
contradicted by it. It was the hope expressed there that
midwives, the main professional body concerned with
breastfeeding, would take the lead in establishing a
working party (which would include broad representation
from other bodies) in order to ascertain what the current
evidence suggested was good practice, to which members
of the RCM Council have responded.

The principal members of the working group were
Chloe Fisher (Senior Midwife, Oxford), Sally Garforth
(Midwife, Reading), Sally Inch (Midwife, Oxford, who
has acted as chief editor), Ellena Salariya (Research
Midwife, Dundee) and Michael Woolridge (Research
Fellow, Department of Child Health, Bristol). Jean Rowe
(Health Visitor, London) and Margaret Kerr (Midwife,
Northern Ireland) also contributed to the final document.

The group gratefully acknowledges the help and advice
received from Evelyn Elliott (NCT), Rachel O'Leary
(LLL) and Peggy Thomas (ABM) who attended most of
the working group's meetings; and Phillipa Cardale,
(RCM Serving Officer for the group) who tactfully and
efficiently administered the group.

Thanks are due to all those who read and commented
on the various drafts of the handbook, or otherwise
assisted with its production: *Belinda Ackerman, Ruth
Ashton, David Baum, Joyce Beak, Margaret Bourne,*

V

Margaret Brain, Tricia Brinton, Mary Broadhurst, Margaret Brown, Katherine Caldwell, Iain Chalmers, Petra Clark, Hanna Corbishley, Esther Culpin, Jean Cushing, Eleanor Donachie, Sheila Drayton, Elizabeth Duffin, Carol Files, Caroline Flint, Sheila Fleming, Eunice Foster, Joan Greenwood, Fiona Haines, Gillian Harris, Pauline Henry, Edmund Hey, Mary Hews, Peter Howie, Laura Jones, Joan Jordan, Jean Keats, Mavis Kirkham, Judy Levi, Jean Martin, Dorothy McDonald, Maureen Minchin, Tricia Murphy-Black, Yvonne Peters, June Reed, Mary Renfrew, Anne Rider, Jill Roberts, Wendy Robinson, Patti Rundall, Shirleyanne Seal, James Sikorski, Jacky Simmonds, Alison Spiro, Ann Stewart, Margaret Taylor, Mary Uprichard, Barbara Weller, Brian Wharton, Margaret Williams, Jane Winship, and particularly *Anne Bent,* for her help in editing the penultimate draft.

Reference

1. 'Difficulties with breastfeeding — midwives in disarray?' Report of the 11th Meeting of the Royal Society of Medicine's Forum on Maternity and the Newborn 1987 In: Journal of the Royal Society of Medicine 80: 53–58

Contents

1 **Understanding how a baby breastfeeds** 1

Milk production and the role of lactational hormones.
Milk release and infant 'sucking'.
Changes in the breast during pregnancy and parturition.

2 **Duration and frequency of feeds** 9

Duration of feeds.
Frequency of feeds.
Variability in intake/infant appetite.

3 **Correct positioning of the baby on the breast** 13

Introduction.
The different appearances of breast and bottle feeding.
When to offer help to the mother.
Steps to achieving correct positioning.
Indications that the baby is properly attached.
Ways in which the midwife can help directly.
Postural considerations.
   — Suggestions for the first feed.
   — Helping the mother to feed lying down.
   — Helping the mother to feed sitting up.
   — Position and posture of the midwife.

4 **Factors which have been shown to help** 25

Advice and support at the first feed.
Unrestricted feeds.
   — Unrestricted duration of feeds.
   — Unrestricted frequency of feeds.
Feeding the baby at night.
   — The value of night feeds.
   — Rooming in.
   — Bedding in.
   — Sleep and the mother.

Monitoring the baby's health and
wellbeing.
— Weight.
— Weight gain.
— Weight variations.
— Stools.
— General health.

5 **Factors which have been shown to be
unhelpful** 41
Additional fluids for breastfed babies.
— Dehydration.
— Jaundice.
— Hazards of additional fluids.
Test weighing.
Maternal dietary modifications.
— Additional fluids for breastfeeding
mothers.
— Additional calories for breastfeeding
mothers.
— Dietary prohibitions for breastfeeding
mothers.
— Provision of free samples to mothers.
— Promotion of breastmilk substitutes.

6 **Antenatal and postnatal considerations** 53
Influencing the decision to breastfeed.
— Antenatal classes.
Sustaining the decision to breastfeed.
Prevention of feeding problems.
— Antenatal preparation.
— Nipple shape.
— Nipple preparation.
— Expression of colostrum.
Postnatal care of the breasts.
— Cleanliness.
— Creams and ointments.
— Limiting sucking time.
Treatment of sore nipples.
— Resting and expressing.
— Re-positioning.
— Nipple shields.
Prevention and treatment of
engorgement.

Successful breastfeeding

— Vascular engorgement.
— Milk engorgement
— Prevention.
— Treatment.
Prevention and treatment of mastitis.
  — Non-infective mastitis.
  — Infective mastitis.
  — Prevention of non-infective mastitis.
  — Prevention of infective mastitis.
  — Treatment of mastitis.

7 Notes on less common problems 69
Baby vomiting blood.
Blood in milk/colostrum.
Blanching of the nipple (white nipple).
Thrush infection of the nipple.
Contact dermatitis.
Diabetes.
Epilepsy.
Anticoagulant therapy.
Other drugs and breastfeeding.
Mammary surgery.
Cleft lip.
Cleft palate.
Down's syndrome.
Tandem feeding.
Breast abscess.
Inverted nipples.
AIDS and breastfeeding.
Herpes simplex infection.

8 Breastfeeding under special circumstances 75
Preterm infants.
  — HIV and milk banking.
Caesarean section.
Twins.
Triplets.
Establishing lactation with an electric
  pump.
Babies being cared for in units other than
  maternity units.

9 Appendix 1 Voluntary Organizations 81
National: National Childbirth Trust

Twins and Multiple Births
    Association
La Leche League
Baby Milk Action Coalition
Association of Breastfeeding
    Mothers
International: Geneva Infant Feeding
    Association
International Baby Food
    Action Network
Action for Corporate
    Accountability
La Leche League
    International
International Organisation
    of Consumer Unions
Nursing Mothers' Association
    of Australia.

Appendix 2   Further reading   83

Index   85

Successful breastfeeding

Introduction

This handbook has been written to help midwives, and others, provide more effective advice and support for the breastfeeding women in their care.

Human milk has evolved over many thousands of years to meet the specific needs of human infants; just as the milk of all other mammals has evolved to meet the specific needs of their young. Not surprisingly therefore, the more that is known about the nutritional, immunological and other properties of breast milk, the more superior it appears in comparison with all other available milks for human babies. Thus it is regarded as axiomatic, in this handbook, that unless individual circumstances make it impossible, all babies should be exclusively breastfed until they are at least four, and preferably six months old. No attempt is made to list the specific benefits, which are well documented elsewhere (1, 2, 3, 4–10).

The majority of women in Great Britain (64%) now choose to breastfeed (5). In spite of this only a few (26%) are still fully breastfeeding at four months, which is the minimum duration recommended at the time these data were compiled (6).

Many women abandon breastfeeding during the first two weeks (5) when midwifery care is still intensive. The World Health Organization have accepted that the vast majority of women (97% or more) are physiologically capable of breastfeeding their babies successfully (7). The discrepancy between those who are capable and those who succeed may pinpoint weaknesses among those who support them rather than the women themselves. Indeed one Australian writer attributes a large part of the responsibility for breastfeeding failure to professional ignorance (8). She continues:

I am not imputing negligence or stupidity or malice, or making any other moral judgements. I know that most professionals are hard working, humane and dedicated. I am reporting that there is a degree of professional ignorance which is historically quite understandable, but no longer tolerable.

Teaching a mother breastfeeding skills may lack the glamour and urgency of intrapartum care, but it is an integral, and can be an equally rewarding, part of a midwife's role. Furthermore the midwife, as the key health worker in the early postnatal days, has the opportunity and privilege of making a tremendous difference to the experience and success of breastfeeding women.

However, every woman who has started to breastfeed her baby and every midwife who has tried to help, will be familiar with the widespread experience of conflicting advice, to which the Report of the Maternity Services Advisory Committee (9) has recently drawn attention. It is hoped that this handbook will overcome the conflict in the advice given to breastfeeding women, as it bases its recommendations for practice on sound research evidence.

The need to achieve consistency and rationality in the support given by midwives and other staff is even more important in view of the difficulties imposed by the present system of care. Ideally, a mother and her baby would receive all their care from one skilled individual. However, most women now have their babies in a hospital where there is shift system of staff for postnatal care.

This is compounded by the present economic restraints within the health service which often results in a midwife being responsible for as many as 30 mothers and babies at a time. Consequently the time available to help each individual woman establish breastfeeding is severely restricted. It is therefore crucial that the advice and support that midwives can offer is the best available and that it is constantly reinforced by all their colleagues.

The needs of the baby have been adequately met, in most cases, by the intricate physiological mechanisms of the mother's body during the months spent in utero. The mother's breasts can provide a fluid that is equally intricate, and precisely tailored to the baby's extra-uterine needs. No other food can match it and the possible short- and long-term consequences of depriving babies of breastmilk are only just beginning to be investigated. In recognition of the importance of breastfeeding to both mothers and babies, this handbook is offered as both a resource and a practical guide for midwives.

It begins with a brief outline of the history of breastfeeding in Britain this century, and thus an explanation for the fact that so many midwives find themselves ill-equipped to assist breastfeeding women. The remainder of the handbook is consequently devoted to providing sound, research based information to increase their knowledge, skill and confidence.

The first section explains the physiology of breastfeeding, as a thorough understanding of this is vital for effective care. This is followed by a detailed description of how to position a baby at the breast correctly, as this basic midwifery skill is fundamental to breastfeeding success.

Many of the issues in breastfeeding practice, such as the regulation of feeds or the use of supplementary fluids are then examined in the light of current research findings. Practices which have been shown to help women breastfeed are recommended, and those which may hinder success are identified.

Finally it is recognised that problems and special circumstances do occur. Where appropriate the origins of common problems are discussed, along with effective prevention and treatment.

NOTE: *1. We acknowledge that babies are either male or female, but as all mothers are female, we have, for the sake of clarity, referred to the baby as he or him throughout.*
2. Unless otherwise stated, it should be assumed that the baby is a healthy term infant.

References

Introduction

1. Garza C, Schanler RJ, Butte NF, Motil KJ 1987 Special Properties of Human Milk. Clinics in Perinatology 14(1): 11–32
2. Minchin M 1985 Breastfeeding Matters. Allen & Unwin, Australia, pp. 6–36. (This book is available in the UK from The National Childbirth Trust. See Appendix 1.) See also Minchin M 1987 Infant Formula: A Mass Uncontrolled Trial in Perinatal Care. Birth 14: 97–100
3. Riordan J, Countryman B 1983 The Biological Specificity of Breastmilk. In: Riordan J (ed.) A Practical Guide to Breastfeeding. CVMosby, St. Louis. pp. 28–39
4. American Academy of Pediatrics Committee on Nutrition 1978 Paediatrics 62: 591
5. Infant Feeding 1985 OPCS Social Survey Division
6. DHSS 1974 Report on Health and Social Subjects No. 9 Present day

Practice in Infant Feeding. HMSO, London
and:
DHSS 1980 Report on Health and Social Subjects No. 20 HMSO, London
and:
DHSS 1988 Report on Health and Social Subjects No. 32 Present day Practice in Infant Feeding. HMSO, London

7. Chetley A 1986 The Politics of Babyfood – Successful Challenges to an International Marketing Strategy. Francis Pinter (In which he quotes the World Health Organization's provisional summary record of the 8th meeting of Committee A, 33rd World Health Assembly; Document No. A33/A SR/8; Geneva, 17th May 1980, p. 11)

8. Minchin M 1985 op. cit. (Breastfeeding Matters) pp. 44–45

9. Maternity Care in Action 1985 Report of the Maternity Services Advisory Committee Part 3. Care of Mother & Baby (Postnatal and neonatal care) p. 5

10. Howie P et al 1990 Protective effect of breastfeeding against infection. British Medical Journal 300: 11–16

Successful breastfeeding

The background

Around the year 1900, concern was growing about the future of the British race. The unacceptably high infant mortality rate was thought to be the result of two major factors: artificial feeding (1) and the 'ignorance and fecklessness of mothers' (2).

The medical profession's response to this was to try to make artificial feeding 'scientific' and therefore safe. There followed a short but intense period of interest in the composition and preparation of bottle feeds; and a small number of doctors emerged as 'experts' on infant feeding, about which they wrote prolifically. Unfortunately their books also contained much advice about breastfeeding, a subject on which it was thought that they would be equally knowledgeable.

Two ideas originated at this time, neither of which appears to have been seriously questioned subsequently. The first was that the breastfed baby fed from the nipple, as if it were a teat on a bottle, rather than from the breast.

Breastfeeding was thus thought to be a traumatic process and mothers were strongly advised to restrict the duration of feeds in the first few days in order to prevent nipple damage. The other idea, which may have originated in Europe, was that severe digestive disorders were likely to be the result of overfeeding breastfed babies. The medical 'experts' thus invented rules relating to the frequency with which a baby should be fed, in order to prevent these conditions. The breastfeeding rules appeared in text books so often that they soon became widely accepted practices, on the assumption that they were scientifically based. These ideas were also disseminated in the 'schools' that were set up for the 'ignorant' mothers.

At this time most women were giving birth at home and they continued to breastfeed as they had always done, with their friends and relatives supporting, advising and handing down the art of breastfeeding. Wealthy women, however, gave birth in nursing homes and hospitals under the care of doctors, and were thus taught the new rules. Coincidentally, medical writers began to comment on the inability of upper class women to breastfeed successfully, a fact which they attributed to the effects of 'higher civilisation' (3). Within a few years of their origin, the rigid rules had become firmly established in most hospitals, and more women were exposed to them as hospital births increased.

By the 1960s, when breastfeeding levels reached an all time low, most women were giving birth in hospital.

Dried cows' milk, which was produced for the government during the Second World War as an alternative, readily available method of infant feeding, continued to be supplied cheaply – or even free – by the newly formed welfare state, as National Dried Milk; and this may also have contributed to the decreased incidence of breastfeeding. As fewer and fewer mothers breastfed, both mothers and midwives lost their skills in the art of breastfeeding.

Because of changes both in society and the place of birth, many families do not now have continuous, consistent support from relatives and neighbours. For this reason many women are more dependent on midwives for support than ever before. It is thus of the utmost importance, both for the sake of the women in their care and for the sake of the profession, that midwives strive to improve their knowledge of, and skills in, breastfeeding. It is the one part of their role which can be said to belong, undeniably, to them.

References

Background
1. Howarth WJ 1905 The Influence of Feeding on Mortality of Infants. Lancet ii: 210–13
2. Lewis J 1980 The Politics of Motherhood. Croom Helm. p. 61.
3. Vincent R 1904 The Nutrition of the Infant. Bailliere, Tindall & Cox, London. p. 32

Successful breastfeeding

Understanding how a baby breastfeeds

Milk production and the role of lactational hormones   1
Milk release and infant 'sucking'   3
Changes in the breast during pregnancy and parturition   6

Milk production and the role of lactational hormones

Milk is produced by the glandular epithelial cells within the breast and is stored in small clusters of '*sac-like*' spaces (alveoli). Around each sac is a basket array of muscle (myoepithelial) cells. Adequate milk production depends on two main factors: (i) prolactin release from the anterior pituitary, which stimulates milk manufacture, and (ii) oxytocin release from the posterior pituitary, which causes the myoepithelial cells to contract, allowing the manufactured and stored milk to be released. The milk drains into the 10–15 '*ampullae*', or lactiferous sinuses, which lie behind the nipple, and removal from here is effected by the rhythmical pressure exerted by the baby's tongue (see p. 5). The effective functioning of both aspects of milk production is accomplished in the majority of women by means of the unrestricted and efficient suckling of the baby.

The level of prolactin in the maternal bloodstream rises steadily during pregnancy, but milk production cannot begin until the placental steroid hormones, progesterone and oestrogen, have declined (following the delivery of the placenta) to the point where they no longer inhibit the action of prolactin. (Very rarely, retained placental fragments may prevent this decline (1).) The length of time between placental delivery and milk synthesis varies, but seems generally to be between 48 and 96 hours.

In response to appropriate stimuli, initially from suckling, nervous impulses are carried to the posterior pituitary and, by an unconditioned reflex, cause the release of oxytocin into the maternal bloodstream. This subsequently affects all the oxytocin receptors in the mother's body, including those in the uterus, causing the characteristic '*afterpains*' often associated with early breastfeeding, particularly in multiparous women. Later, oxytocin may be released by a conditioned reflex in response to the sight or sound of the baby, or as a result of preparation for breastfeeding. There is no evidence that the *unconditioned* reflex can be inhibited by anxiety.

Once lactation is established, its continued success seems to depend rather less on high levels of prolactin, and rather more on the efficient removal of milk from the alveolar sacs. As one writer has said: 'Drainage, not milk production, is the sine qua non of successful breastfeeding.' (2).

Efficient milk removal can be impaired, and lactation adversely affected, if the breasts are allowed to become engorged (see p. 61). In this situation the alveoli become so full that the myoepithelial cells are unable to contract strongly enough to expel the milk (3).

The '*let-down*' or milk ejection reflex (in response to oxytocin release) is highly variable. In some women it is extremely vigorous, causing sharp, needle-like pains in the breast, and if the ducts are open at the nipple surface, milk may spurt out in jets. Other mothers experience a tingling sensation, and milk may only drip from the breast. At the other extreme, some mothers may experience no sensation at all, but as long as the myoepithelial cells contract sufficiently to create a positive pressure in the duct system, milk will be brought down into the lactiferous ducts where it can be stripped from the breast by the action of the baby's mouth and tongue.

This variability seems to reflect differences in maternal physiology (4), but all these responses are normal.

Some babies appear to ingest only the milk which is ejected by the mother, taking hardly any by their own efforts. In an otherwise neurologically normal baby, this is likely to be due to early mismanagement of breastfeeding. Clinical experience suggests that unless the baby's feeding technique is improved by better positioning, milk production will decline to below his needs.

Babies of mothers with poorly developed milk ejection must derive all their milk by actively stripping milk from the breast. For this group, correct attachment and positioning at the breast is also vital for effective milk removal.

It is worth stressing that breastmilk (unlike a breastmilk substitute) is not uniform in composition. During the feed the fat (and hence the calorie) content rises as the rate of milk flow declines (see p. 28). This makes it very difficult to state which stage of the feed is the most nutritious. In fact the different stages are nutritious in different ways. Changes in feed management can affect the balance of nutrients taken by the baby in both the short and the long term. For this reason, arbitrary rules for breastfeeding management should not be imposed.

Milk release and infant sucking

Milk is transferred from the breast to the baby by a combination of two processes: (i) active milk expulsion by the mother due to her let-down reflex, and (ii) active removal by the baby who, by working on the tissues of the breast with jaw and tongue, strips milk from the milk ducts (5). Both processes are necessary to ensure that the infant obtains both the full volume and the full nutrient content of the feed.

Much can be done to promote the first of these by encouraging the mother in her efforts to breastfeed and imbuing her with confidence in her ability to feed. This is no small task, and teaching the mother good breastfeeding technique is fundamental to these aims.

To strip the milk efficiently from the breast, both the baby and the mother must be taught what constitutes effective attachment at the breast. The mother needs to learn to make use of her baby's natural reflexes. To start with, the baby should be facing the mother's breast, so that his neck is neither twisted nor flexed (6). Brushing the baby's lips against the nipple will trigger the rooting reflex (7), the most important component of which is that, if encouraged correctly in the early days, the baby's mouth will gape wide to accept the breast (see Figs 1, 2 and 3).

The wider the baby's gape, the easier it will be for the mother to attach her baby to her breast effectively. It is therefore important for the mother to draw a strong response from her baby in the early days (see p. 19) .

In some cases, correct attachment may be made easier if the mother forms

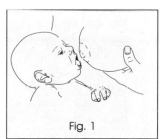

Fig. 1

3

her breast, (including the nipple, areola and underlying tissue) into an appropriate shape by supporting it from underneath. With a positive action, by moving her baby onto the breast, this is positioned within the baby's mouth. The mother should not push her nipple towards the baby (8).

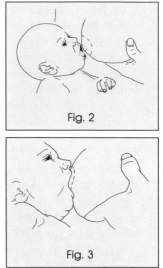

Fig. 2

Fig. 3

The process by which the baby removes milk from the breast is analogous to hand milking the teats of a cow's udder, whereby milk is expressed from the teat by a rhythmical rolling action of the fingers against the palm of the hand. During breastfeeding, the baby's tongue does the equivalent job of the fingers. It must be stressed that because it is the tongue which works on the lactiferous sinuses, the relationship between these two components is crucial to good feeding. Consequently, locating the lower jaw well away from the base of the nipple is the first step to ensuring correct attachment (9) (see Fig. 4). The mother's nipple will extend back to the soft palate if the baby is correctly attached to the breast. This stimulation of the sucking reflex (10, 11) causes: (i) the baby's lower jaw to clamp onto the breast tissue, (ii) suction to be exerted, thus holding the nipple well into the mouth, and (iii) rhythmical cycles of compression to be applied by the tongue to the teat-like shape formed from the breast and the nipple, squeezing milk from the ducts. The 'teat' lies in a furrow formed by the tongue, and the wave of compression moves back along this trough, from the breast to the baby, occluding it and forcing milk from the ampullae within the teat.

Milk will remain available for removal as long as a pressure gradient remains in the milk ducts. This is created both by positive pressure in the alveoli, due to myoepithelial contraction, and negative pressure outside the nipple, from the baby's mouth.

4

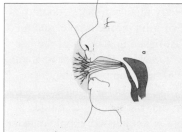

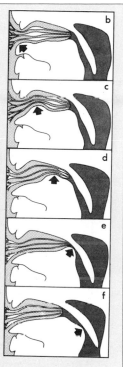

Fig. 4: Shows a complete 'suck' cycle. The baby is shown in median section, and exhibits good feeding technique with the nipple drawn well into the mouth, extending back to the junction of the hard and soft palate. (The lactiferous sinuses are depicted within the teat, though these cannot be visualised on scans.)

a. A 'teat' is formed from the nipple and much of the areola, with the lacteal sinuses, (which lie behind the nipple) being drawn into the mouth with the breast tissue. The soft palate is relaxed and the nasopharynx is open for breathing. The shape of the tongue at the back represents its position at rest, cupped around the tip of the nipple.

b. The suck cycle is initiated by the welling up of the anterior of the tongue. At the same time, the lower jaw, which had been momentarily relaxed (not shown) is raised to constrict the base of the nipple, thereby 'pinching off' milk within the ducts of the teat (these movements are inferred as they lie outside the sector viewed in ultrasound scans).

c. The wave of compression by the tongue, moves along the underside of the nipple in a posterior direction, pushing against the hard palate. This roller-like action squeezes milk from the nipple. The posterior position of the tongue may be depressed as milk collects in the oropharynx.

d & e. The wave of compression passes back past the tip of the nipple, in a posterior direction, pushing against the soft palate. As the tongue impinges on the soft palate the levator muscles of the palate contract, raising it to seal off the nasal cavity. Milk is pushed into the oropharynx and is swallowed if sufficient has collected.

f. The cycle of compression continues and ends at the posterior base of the tongue. Depression of the back portion of the tongue creates negative pressure, drawing the nipple and its milk contents back into the mouth. This is accompanied by a lowering of the jaw, which allows milk to flow back into the nipple.

In ultrasound scans it appears that compression by the tongue, and negative pressure with the mouth, maintain the tongue in close conformation to the nipple and palate. Events are portrayed here rather more loosely to aid clarity.

Understanding how a baby breastfeeds

If the baby is correctly attached, there should be no friction of the tongue or gum on the nipple, and no movement of the breast tissue in and out of the baby's mouth. Thus the baby's sucking should not traumatise the nipple, and there should be no soreness. Pain is a biological warning signal, and in the context of breastfeeding is a sign that the feeding technique is imperfect. If this signal is not heeded, nipple damage will result. Figures 5 and 6 illustrate incorrect positioning, and Figures 7 and 8 illustrate correct positioning.

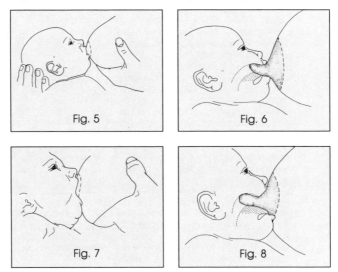

Fig. 5

Fig. 6

Fig. 7

Fig. 8

Changes in the breast during pregnancy and parturition

The changes in the breast during pregnancy are documented in most well referenced books on the breast and breastfeeding (12, 13). As far as changes relevant to their efficiency for breastfeeding, attention has been focused in the past on the adequacy of the mother's nipples. There is little evidence to suggest that there is anything to be gained by antenatal assessment or preparation of the mother's nipples (see pp. 56–57).

The most dramatic changes in nipple shape take place around parturition and in the early postnatal period (14). Furthermore, with skilled help, babies can be correctly attached to breasts which may be considered to have '*inadequate nipples*' (see also p. 72). There is no justification for informing a mother, on the basis of an antenatal inspection of her nipples, that she may be incapable of breastfeeding. This will only serve to damage her confidence and can be a self-fulfilling prophecy.

References

Milk production and role of lactational hormones

1. Neifert M, McDonough S, Neville M 1981 Failure of Lactogenesis Associated with Placental Retention. American Journal of Obstetrics and Gynecology 140: 477–478
2. Applebaum RM 1970 The Modern Management of Successful Breastfeeding. Pediatric Clinics of North America 17: 203–225
3. Dawson EK 1935 Edinburgh Medical Journal 42: 569
4. Lucas A, Drewett RF, Mitchell MD 1980 Breastfeeding and Plasma Oxytocin Concentrations. British Medical Journal 281: 834–835
5. Woolridge MW 1986 The 'Anatomy' of Infant Sucking. Midwifery 2: 164–171
6. Gunther M 1973 Infant Feeding. Penguin.

Mechanisms of milk release and infant 'sucking'

7. Prechtl HFR 1958 The Directed Head Turning Response and Allied Movements of the Human Baby. Behaviour 13: 212–242
8. Fisher C 1981 Breastfeeding: A Midwife's View. Maternal and Child Health February: 52–57
9. Woolridge MW 1986 Aetiology of Sore Nipples. Midwifery 2: 172–176
10. Gunther M 1955 Instinct and the Nursing Couple. Lancet i: 575–578
11. Peiper A 1963 Cerebral Function in Infancy and Childhood, 3rd edn. Consultants Bureau, New York. pp. 418–420

Changes in the breast during pregnancy and parturition

12. Vorherr H 1974 The Breast: Morphology, Physiology and Lactation. Academic Press, New York
13. Neville MC, Neifert MR 1983 Lactation: Physiology, Nutrition and Breastfeeding. Plenum, New York
14. Hytten FE, Baird D 1958 The Development of the Nipple in Pregnancy. Lancet i (7032): 1201–1204

Duration and frequency of feeds

Duration of feeds   9
Frequency of feeds   10
Variability in intake/infant appetite   10

Duration of feeds

Recent studies have used electronic weighing scales to attempt to answer the question 'How long should a breastfeed last?' Earlier work had suggested that milk transfer takes place rapidly in the first few minutes of a feed (1). This is now known to be a misleading picture derived by measuring a cross section of babies feeding for different lengths of time. Measuring intake at repeated points during a feed has shown that such a picture does not apply to individual babies (2, 3). For many mothers, milk transfer may take much longer than a few minutes, sometimes occurring very slowly. As with all biological systems there is tremendous variability in the rate at which milk is transferred from mother to baby and in the demand for milk by the baby. However, the general picture that emerges is that, if all other aspects of feeding are ideal, babies take roughly equivalent amounts of milk, but after varying periods of time on the breast (3).

This concept is crucial to the management of breastfeeds. It suggests that babies will normally feed for a length of time that is appropriate to the rate of milk transfer, naturally regulating their intake. Thus a baby who takes milk at a high rate will feed for a short time, whereas if milk transfer occurs at a slow rate the baby will need to feed for much longer. In consequence, it is inappropriate to tell a mother how long a feed should last, and there should be no set rules on the length of feeds at any time in the postnatal period (2).

However, it is important to recognise the circumstances which, if uncorrected, may cause feeds to be unnecessarily long (e.g. regularly more than 30 minutes per breast) as may be the case if the infant is incorrectly positioned at the breast when feeding. Incorrect positioning may result not only in protracted feeds, but may cause nipple damage, the severity of which will be in direct proportion to the length of the feed. The solution in these

9

circumstances is not to restrict the feed length (as this will create other problems – see p. 27), but to improve the positioning. Feeding can then continue without any need for restrictions.

Frequency of feeds

The interval between feeds will determine the number of feeds the baby takes in any 24 hour period. Once again, there are no set rules for either the number or the frequency of feeds that should be given. Some babies will want feeding at intervals of $1^1/_2$–2 hours, while others will go much longer between feeds (4–6 hours); mothers should be reassured that it does not matter if their baby does not appear to be '*typical*'.

When breastfeeding is established, however, feeds that are regularly less than an hour apart may be an indication that the baby is incorrectly positioned at the breast. If this is the case the baby may be unable to consume the high fat hindmilk. The low fat feeds will have a rapid stomach transit time (4, 5) and may result in short intervals between feeds. Thus changes in management, i.e. improving feeding technique, can effect an improvement in other aspects of breastfeeding.

Variability in intake/infant appetite

Lactation is acknowledged to be regulated by the process of supply and demand, most probably with the infant's demand for milk regulating the supply (6). Thus the mother of twins can produce twice as much milk as the mother of one baby, as there is twice the demand (7, 8) (see also p. 77). The amount of milk a baby 'demands' is regulated by appetite, which exerts control over the baby's intake in the same way that an adult's appetite does. This can be demonstrated by the fact that even newborn infants may finish feeding when milk is still available to them in the breast (9).

In order for the infant to regulate his intake according to his needs, he must be allowed to express his appetite fully. To do this he must: (i) be fed on demand (i.e. when he requests) and (ii) be allowed to feed until satiated (i.e. for an unrestricted period of time). Only then can the natural process of appetite control operate, and the baby regulate his intake to suit his individual and changing needs. As every baby's needs differ, the pattern of feeding cannot be predicted, and should not be prescribed (10).

Some mothers may try to restrict their baby's feeds in the belief that it is necessary (and possible) to condition him to go longer between feeds, because they cannot face the prospect of the feeding pattern of the first few weeks continuing for months. All mothers should be reassured that both the frequency and the duration of the feeds tend to decrease with time.

On the other hand, an otherwise healthy baby who is feeding less than six times in 24 hours at the end of the first week may be losing his appetite. Incorrect positioning, and thus an inadequate intake, often results in apathy which is not accompanied by any other signs of illness.

References

The duration of feeds
1. Lucas A, Lucas PJ, Baum JD 1979 Patterns of Milk Flow in Breastfed Infants. Lancet ii: 57–58
2. Howie PW, Houston MJ, Cook A, Smart L, McArdle F, McNeilly AS 1981 How Long Should a Breast Feed Last? Early Human Development 5: 71–77
3. Woolridge MW, Baum JD, Drewett RF 1982 Individual Patterns of Milk Intake During Breastfeeding. Early Human Development 7: 265–272

Frequency of feeds
4. Spiller RC, Trotman IF, Higgins BE, et al 1984 The Ilial Brake – Inhibition of Jejunal Motility after Ilial Fat Perfusion in Man. Gut 25: 365–374
5. Anonymous 1986 Milk Fat, Diarrhoea and the Ilial Brake. Lancet i: 658

Variability in intake and infant appetite
6. Woolridge MW, Baum JD 1987 The Regulation of Human Milk Flow. In: Lindblad B (ed) 'Perinatal Nutrition' Vol 6, Bristol-Meyers. pp. 243–257 Nutrition Symposia.
   See also:
   Prentice A 1986 Cross Culture Differences in Lactational Performance. In: Hamosh M. Goldman A. (eds) Human Lactation 2. Plenum Press, New York
7. Hartmann PE, Prosser CG 1984 Physiological Basis of Longitudinal Changes in Human Milk Yield and Composition. Federation Proceedings 43/9: 2448–2453
8. Saint L, Maggiore P, Hartmann PE 1986 Yield and Nutrient Content of Milk in 8 Women Breastfeeding Twins and 1 Woman Breastfeeding Triplets. British Journal of Nutrition 56: 49–58

9. Drewett RF, Woolridge MW 1981 Milk Taken by Human Babies from the First and the Second Breast. Physiology and Behaviour 26: 327–329

10. Cran DHD 1913 Breastfeeding: Dr. Variot's Teaching. Lancet i: 1659–1660

Correct positioning of the baby at the breast

Introduction   13
The different appearances of breast and bottle feeding   13
When to offer help to the mother   14
Steps to achieving correct positioning   15
Indications that the baby is properly attached   18
Ways in which the midwife can help directly   19
Postural considerations   20

Introduction

A very high proportion of early breastfeeding problems may be due to a failure to position the baby correctly on the breast. When babies are badly positioned, the *'quality'* of the mouthful of breast tissue which the baby takes in may be inadequate for the jaw and tongue to express the milk effectively.

Unfortunately, many of the problems commonly associated with incorrect positioning, such as nipple pain and soreness without overt signs of infection; protracted feeds; a baby that cries hungrily after a feed and *'breastmilk insufficiency'*, are still reported, followed by the statement *'the baby was properly on'*. This suggests that midwives' assessment of what constitutes 'properly on' differ greatly. It is important for midwives to reassess their criteria for making this statement, for it is an issue about which there should be no complacency.

The different appearances of breast and bottle feeding

Industrialised Western society has become unfamiliar with the sight of a mother breastfeeding in public. As a result it may be imagined that the baby with a breast in his mouth should look much the same as a baby with a bottle teat in his mouth (1). This is not the case, as the *'sucking'* action on the breast is mechanically different from that on the bottle (2, 3, 4) (see Figs 9 and 10).

As a demonstration of the difference, try this simple exercise: place a finger in your mouth as if it were a bottle teat, and suck. You will notice that your cheeks cave in as suction is created. Now suck your forearm, so that your

13

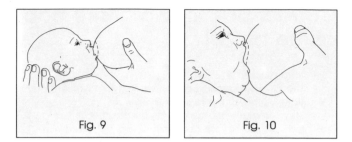

Fig. 9

Fig. 10

mouth is full, as should be the case with breastfeeding. Your mouth and jaw action will be very different, involving all the muscles of your face.

An appreciation of the intrinsic, qualitative difference between breast and bottle feeding is a necessary part of teaching good feeding technique to a mother. Commercial literature suggesting that any teat is similar to the breast should be disregarded (5).

When to offer help to the mother

There are two different circumstances in which the guidelines offered here may be of help to midwives, and it is important to distinguish between them.

A soundly based knowledge of the physiology, together with the skills derived from close observation and familiarity with breastfeeding, should enable all midwives to provide the help and support required by mothers as they begin to breastfeed. Initially, however, this help should consist of verbal instruction only; the midwife should describe the essential features of good feeding technique to the mother and suggest possible ways in which she may improve it.

Only if a mother is unable to achieve a satisfactory feeding technique and clearly needs assistance should the midwife give more direct help. This may also apply if specific problems present themselves at a later stage, in which case the midwife may need to offer active help at this time.

It may be that on occasions professionals intervene too quickly, rather than observing and encouraging the mother's own efforts. However, it should be remembered that 'once the baby (and also the mother) has experienced one satisfactory feed, subsequent feeds should be better' (6). If the midwife feels that the '*satisfactory feed*' can best be achieved with her active help, she should not be afraid to give it.

Steps to achieving correct positioning

1. Whatever the exact orientation of the baby's body relative to his mother's, he should be close to her with his head and shoulders facing her breast. The baby's whole body should be square onto the mother and his nose should be at the same level as the nipple (see Figs. 11, 12, 13 and 14).

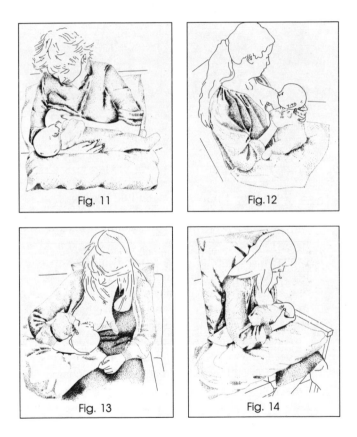

Fig. 11   Fig. 12

Fig. 13   Fig. 14

2. The baby (head, shoulders and trunk) should be moved straight towards the breast with a swift, positive and well directed action. There should be no sudden change of direction such as would be the case with flexion of the head or movement away from the midline of the breast.

15

Correct positioning of the baby at the breast

3. The lower one-third of a baby's gaping mouth is occupied by the tongue, so that if, when the baby is brought onto the breast, the nipple is aimed towards the lower part of the mouth it will simply come up against the tongue. Instead, if the nipple is aimed into the upper third of the mouth it will go past the tongue and drive against the roof of the mouth (see Fig. 15). The baby's tongue will then lie against the breast tissue extending back from the base of the nipple.

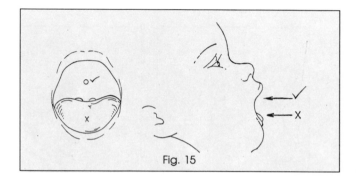

Fig. 15

4. If the baby's nose is pressed into the breast, he may be too high on the breast, causing his neck to become flexed. Moving him lower, while still keeping him close to his mother's body, will ensure that his neck and head are extended and that his nose is free. If the baby is lying horizontally (across his mother's body) his whole body may need to be moved along, feet first, towards the breast that is not being suckled. This will also have the effect of slightly extending his head and neck.

If the head and neck are slightly extended, there will be no need to press the breast away from his nostrils. Doing so tends to pull the nipple back, and may compress the milk sinuses within the breast, thus preventing milk flow. However, hyperextension of the baby's head and neck must also be avoided, as it makes swallowing impossible. If the baby's bottom lies out across the mother's lap, pulling his hips closer in towards the mother's trunk should create a space between nose and mouth.

5. Opinions differ as to which hand should be used for: (i)

supporting and presenting the breast, and (ii) supporting the baby and moving him towards the breast. Mothers (and/or babies) often have a preferred side, and feeding technique may be improved on the less favoured side by using the same hands for the same tasks as on the preferred side. This may entail changing the direction in which the baby lies.

6. Most mothers and babies benefit from the breast being well supported, especially if the mother has large or very elastic breasts. This support can be provided either with the mother's fingers placed flat against her ribs at the base of her breast, or with her hand cupping her breast. In the latter case, her thumb should be on top of her breast, but well away from her nipple, with her remaining four fingers below (see Fig. 16).

It is important that the mother is discouraged from using a 'scissor grip' when offering her breast. This pushes the glandular tissue backwards, preventing the baby from drawing the lactiferous sinuses into his mouth, and the fingers themselves prevent the baby from getting far enough onto the breast.

Fig. 16

7. It is sometimes helpful to tilt a large or elastic breast up as the baby is put on, pointing the nipple towards the roof of his mouth, or even at his nose. This helps to locate his lower lip and jaw well below the nipple.

8. When supporting her baby, the mother should either support the head and shoulders on her forearm, or hold her baby across the shoulders with her free hand, supporting his head with her fingers. She should be discouraged from holding the back of his head with her hand, as this may cause him distress, particularly if his head is forced onto the breast.

17

Correct positioning of the baby at the breast

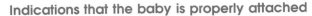

3

Indications that the baby is properly attached

1. If the baby is properly attached, his mouth will be wide open and the lower lip will be further away from the base of the nipple than the top lip (see Fig. 17). The bottom lip will curl back *automatically* and will be some way from the base of the nipple.

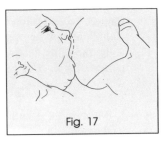

Fig. 17

If the lower lip appears to be pinching at the base of the nipple, the baby is not properly attached.

2. The baby will have a mouth full of breast, which will include the nipple, much of the areola and all the underlying tissue including the milk ducts. This will cause a typical jaw action as the baby works on the breast. The jaw muscles work rhythmically, and this action extends as far back as the ears. If the cheeks are being sucked inwards, the baby is not properly attached.

3. Do not be guided by how much areola can be seen above the baby's top lip, as this gives no indication as to where the tongue and the lower jaw are located. There is much variability between mothers in the size of the areola, and the advice to '*get all the areola into the baby's mouth*' is irrelevant and often impractical.

4. After an initial short burst of sucking the rhythm will be slow and even with deep jaw movements. Pauses are uncommon early in the feed once the milk has started to flow but they become more marked as the feed progresses.

5. The baby will terminate the feed of his own accord by coming off the breast spontaneously. A baby is able to express satiety, as well as hunger, by his behaviour.

18

Ways in which the midwife can help directly

One of the most important things you should do is to describe what you are doing, and why you are doing it.

1. Hold the baby with the heel of your hand behind his shoulders, with your fingers supporting his head.

2. It may be helpful, when the breast is large or soft, to 'firm' it by applying gentle pressure with the other hand, placing your thumb below and your fingers on top.

3. Move the baby against the breast, teasing him by brushing his upper lip against the nipple. Wait until he begins to open his mouth wide before moving him onto the breast.

4. When you are confident that he will open his mouth widely, and the moment that you see the lower lip start to drop, move him onto the breast quickly with a positive but gentle action (see Fig. 18).

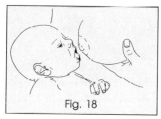

Fig. 18

5. Aim the baby's bottom jaw as far away from the base of the nipple as possible, so that he gets as much of the breast in his mouth as he can. He must get far enough onto the breast so that he can squeeze milk out of the ducts behind the areola with his tongue (see Fig. 19). Do not tip his head forward, but move the whole baby towards the mother, keeping his spine straight and his head slightly extended.

6. It is the baby's lower jaw and tongue that work at the breast, so less of the areola will be visible below the lower lip than above his top lip, and his mouth will appear asymmetrically placed (see Fig. 20). *When you are helping the mother in this way, tell her what you are*

19

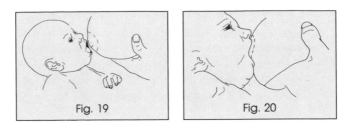

| Fig. 19 | Fig. 20 |

doing and why, and she will then be more likely to achieve it herself.

Many mothers use forceful terms to describe the way in which their baby was handled by helpers, e.g. 'my baby was "*rammed*" onto my breast'. It is not necessary to force the baby onto the breast, and unnecessary pressure on the back of the baby's head can be very distressing to both mother and baby. A sensitive hold and skilled timing are the hallmarks of good practice.

Postural considerations

Suggestions for the first feed

The mother's physical comfort when breastfeeding is important. She may be inclined to overlook any personal discomfort while focusing her attention on the needs of her baby.

Before assisting the mother with the feed it may be appropriate to offer a bed pan, a fresh sanitary pad or more general toileting. The midwife should explain the importance of being comfortable for this and all subsequent feeds.

Such preparation should be made in good time, before the baby is crying hungrily for a feed, as a crying baby cannot easily take the breast. Similarly, the mother should be told that it is not essential to change her baby's nappy before he goes to the breast. (A baby should never be allowed to become distressed before the breast is offered.)

The mother may have definite views about the position she wishes to adopt for feeding, and this must be respected. However, positions which are appropriate for later feeding sessions may not be for the early feeds, particularly if the mother has perineal or abdominal sutures, or has received an epidural or spinal anaesthetic.

The following position for feeding is described in

20

detail, as it is likely to be comfortable for the mother, baby and midwife, particularly for the first few feeds.

Helping the mother to feed lying down

This position is a useful one in which to help the mother. The difficulty with it for the mother is that she may be unable to use the arm on which she is lying to help put her baby to the breast. She should be encouraged to use her free hand to bring the baby towards her, rather than use it to try and put the breast into his mouth (see Fig. 21).

The midwife should recognise that she probably has a preference for helping on one particular side, and unless the mother needs specific help with one breast, she should opt for that side. The midwife may have only one or two opportunities to help a particular woman. The more competent she is, the more confidence she will give the mother (see Fig. 22).

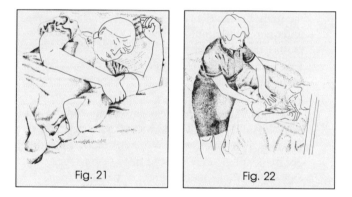

Fig. 21   Fig. 22

The mother should be asked to lie on her side, with her head supported by pillows. If lying on her left side, her left arm should be flexed, with her forearm parallel with her head. She may need a pillow in the small of her back, and one between her knees, for added comfort and support.

The baby should be placed beside and facing the mother, so that he can make eye contact with her. He should not be wrapped in a blanket, so that his hands and feet can make contact with her. The bed clothes should be tucked loosely round the baby and under the mattress, to ensure warmth and safety.

21

Correct positioning of the baby at the breast

Allow time for the mother and baby to interact. The mother may speak to and stroke her baby, or give him her finger to hold. The baby's rooting reflex may be stimulated by the tactile and olfactory sensations he receives.

The mother may comment that the baby appears hungry, but if she does not, the midwife should indicate to her that the baby seems ready to feed.

The baby should be guided gently towards the breast and the mother helped, if necessary, to position him correctly at the breast (see pp. 15–18).

If the midwife has helped to attach the baby, the mother should be encouraged to place her free hand where the midwife's was, once the baby is correctly positioned. Provided the safety of the mother and baby is assured, the midwife can then withdraw a little, unless the mother needs further help, for example to put the baby to the other breast (see Fig. 23).

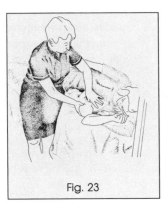

Fig. 23

If the mother experiences correct attachment at the first feed, it is unlikely that she will tolerate incorrect attachment at later feeds. While the mother's and baby's bodily positions may change from feed to feed, the technique of attachment remains the same.

Helping the mother to feed sitting up

In most Western societies, the traditional position for breastfeeding has been sitting upright on a nursing chair. Such chairs were of an appropriate height and had no arm rests. However modern furniture does not always lend itself to good breastfeeding positioning. Often it is too soft, has obstructive armrests and/or sloping backs. Hospital beds and backrests which encourage the mother to lean back are similarly unhelpful.

To achieve correct positioning of the baby at the breast while seated, the mother should be encouraged to lean forwards slightly, so that the breast also falls forward,

22

facilitating attachment. Leaning back flattens the breast, making it much more difficult.

She may need additional pillows to support her back or arms, or raise the baby to a more comfortable level (see Figs. 24 and 25).

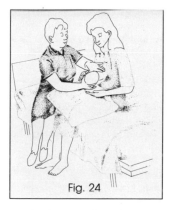

Fig. 24

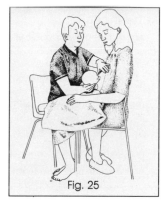

Fig. 25

Having attached the baby correctly, the mother can then be encouraged to relax her back and shoulders against the supporting chair. A footstool may also be a useful aid to relaxation.

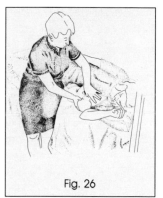

Fig. 26

Position and posture of the midwife

Many midwives experience backache and other

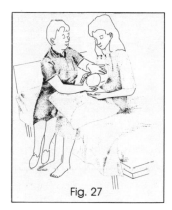

Fig. 27

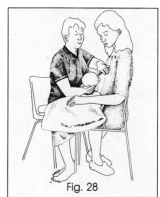

Fig. 28

Correct positioning of the baby at the breast

discomforts when assisting mothers with breastfeeding. It is important that midwives consider their own comfort as well as that of the mother, and avoid positions which will put undue strain on their muscles (see Figs. 26, 27 and 28).

References

Different appearances of breast and bottle feeding

1. Fisher C 1981 Breastfeeding: A Midwife's View. Maternal and Child Health February: 52–57
2. Ardran GM, Kemp FH, Lind J 1958 A Cineradiographic Study of Bottle Feeding. British Journal of Radiology 31: 11–22
3. Ardran GM, Kemp FH, Lind J 1958 A Cineradiographic Study of Breastfeeding. British Journal of Radiology 31: 156–162
4. Woolridge MW 1986 The 'Anatomy' of Infant Sucking. Midwifery 2: 164–171

When to offer help to the mother

5. Minchin M 1985 Breastfeeding Matters. Alma Publication, Allen & Unwin, Australia. Ch 3 & 9
6. Gunther M 1945 Sore Nipples: Causes and Prevention. Lancet ii 590–593

Factors which have been shown to help

4

Advice and support at the first feed   25
Unrestricted feeds   27
Feeding the baby at night   30
Monitoring the baby's health and wellbeing   33

Advice and support at the first feed

The psychological impact on the mother of her first breastfeeding experiences is of undoubted importance. A woman who has just given birth will attach great significance to the way her baby reacts to her and this may affect her feelings towards her baby. A successful first feed is likely to make the mother feel that her baby likes her, and this may be crucial to the continuance of breastfeeding in either the short or the long term (1).

In the past, midwives encouraged suckling soon after the birth, because they recognised the benefit with regard to placental delivery. There may be other benefits conferred by early suckling, as yet undiscovered, and work continues in relation to this.

Researchers in Dundee (2) randomly assigned mothers to different breastfeeding regimes relating to the timing of the first and subsequent feeds. The mothers were followed up for 18 months, at which time the researchers were able to conclude that babies who were first fed within 30 minutes of birth were likely to remain breastfed for longer. Smaller controlled studies in the United States (3), Sweden (4) and Canada (5) which combined early contact and early suckling, support these findings. They also noted that early contact positively affected the behaviour of mothers towards their babies.

Although the benefits of early feeding and early contact have been well documented, controversy still exists as to whether it is the early contact per se or the early suckling which contributes to the extended feeding period. A recent study conducted in Thailand (6) suggests that the quality of the contact may also be important. Mothers who have been separated from their babies soon after delivery

25

should be reassured that high quality contact may be equally valuable whenever it is offered.

It is the midwife's responsibility to ensure that each mother has a satisfactory first feed, as soon as both mother and baby are ready. This will certainly be within 2 hours of birth, in the recognised period of early responsiveness. In most cases the baby will be ready to feed (as distinct from other forms of close contact) within the first hour after birth (7). Yet in recent observations of labour ward practices, carried out in eight health districts in England as part of the 'Policy and Practice in Midwifery' study (8), researchers found that the average time that elapsed between a normal birth and the first feed was 98 minutes; which suggests that some feeds were being unnecessarily delayed. Furthermore they found that in only 44% of cases was a midwife involved with the feed.

Even though the standard delivery bed is not designed to accommodate more than one person, infants may safely experience their first feed while still in the delivery room, provided reasonable care is taken and delivery staff are skilled in helping.

Breastfeeding is a skill to be learned and practised. Many mothers have never seen anyone breastfeeding, and although breastfeeding is natural, it is not instinctive (9). Even multiparous women may need help to get started, particularly if they have never breastfed before, or have had previous difficulties. It is the midwife's responsibility to impart the necessary information about breastfeeding, but whether this is done at the first feed or later as an integral part of the mother's postnatal education, must be decided on an individual basis.

The psychological component of successful breastfeeding should not be underestimated. Midwives, in their supporting role as breastfeeding experts, should reassure the mother that her breasts and nipples are anatomically suitable for the purpose of breastfeeding (unless this is inappropriate) and reinforce her success with praise.

It is hoped that midwives will develop a standardised policy within their workplace in relation to the giving of essential breastfeeding information and, where appropriate, the organising of breastfeeding demonstrations. A policy exists in most health authorities to ensure that all bottle feeding mothers are instructed in the making up of formula feeds and the sterilisation of bottles. The giving of breastfeeding advice should also be regarded as an integral part of the midwife's responsibility for postnatal education, and should be given equal priority.

Appropriate teaching at the first or later feeds will include some or all of the following information:

The composition of colostrum and mature milk should be explained to the mother, who will then understand why her breastfed baby does not require the large volumes given to bottle-fed babies in the first few days of life. She should be told that colostrum is unique and meets the newborn baby's requirements completely, provided the baby has unrestricted access to the breast.

From the very first feed the mother needs to know the importance of correct positioning, as well as being shown how to achieve it.

The physiology of lactation needs to be outlined, using the feed itself to explain: i) the 'let down' of milk, and (ii) the mechanism of milk removal. Explaining the baby's sucking rhythm helps the mother to understand that the pauses are an integral part of the feed and that there is no need to stimulate the baby to suck continuously.

The mother will need to know about her baby's probable feeding needs during the early postnatal period. Information concerning the variable composition of the milk he will receive during a feed, i.e. the graded change from foremilk to hindmilk, will help her to appreciate that she should not attempt to restrict the duration of his feeds.

She should also be told that there may be periods, as the baby grows, when the feeding frequency may increase for a day or so. It is thought that this is the baby's way of ensuring that the milk supply remains adequate for his increasing needs.

Unrestricted feeds

Unrestricted duration of feeds

For many years there has been a widespread belief that it is necessary to limit sucking time, particularly in the early days, in order to prevent sore nipples (10–12) (see also

27

section 6 on the postnatal prevention of feeding problems). Recent studies have shown that nipple soreness is not affected by the duration of the feed (13, 14). Unfortunately the advice to a mother to limit her baby's suckling time, at either or both breast(s) will not only do no good, it will in many cases do harm (15, 16). It has been known for some time that the composition and rate of flow of milk from the human breast changes in composition as the feed progresses (17). The result is that at the start of the feed the baby takes a large volume of low calorie foremilk, changing to a small volume of high calorie hindmilk at the end of the feed (18). It has also been shown that babies will feed at the breast for very different lengths of time if left undisturbed, and that the length of feed is probably determined by the rate of milk transfer between mother and baby (19) (see p. 9). Thus, although there are many babies who will terminate a feed spontaneously in under 10 minutes, those who have a slow rate of transfer will take longer than this. Even though they may not be consuming large volumes after this time, the milk may be sufficiently high in fat (and therefore calories) to make a significant contribution to the energy value of the feed (20). If the mother believes that she must limit her baby's time at the breast, or that she must use both breasts at each feed (and therefore deliberately removes him from the first breast before he finishes spontaneously) she may be significantly curtailing her baby's calorie intake. In such situations the baby may fail to gain weight despite frequent feeds and an apparently good supply of milk (21).

Over-production of milk, causing discomfort and distress, may also be a consequence of limiting feeds, as the baby seeks to compensate for his reduced calorie intake by feeding more frequently, thereby removing large amounts of foremilk which are rapidly replaced (16).

A mother should be encouraged to allow her baby to finish the first breast before offering the second, and should be reassured that it does not matter if her baby only wants to feed from one breast at an individual feed. If she starts with the other breast at the next feed there should be no long term imbalance in milk production. She should be similarly reassured that if her baby requires both breasts at a feed, this is equally acceptable, and that he may shift from one pattern of feeding to another as the volume of milk adjusts to his needs.

Unless the total duration of the feed is very protracted (see p. 9), which may indicate that the mother needs more help to ensure that her baby is correctly positioned, the baby is likely to 'know' better than anyone else for how long (and how often) he needs to be fed.

Unrestricted frequency of feeds

It has already been noted (see p. xv) that the steadily increasing number of women delivered in hospital received the misguided advice that they should regulate the frequency of their baby's feeds.

Gradually, however, careful observations of the unrestricted feeding behaviour of normal infants were made and published (22–24). It became apparent from these and later studies (14, 25) that feeds are usually infrequent for the first day or so, rapidly increase between the 3rd and 7th day and then decrease. It was also found that although some babies with frequencies at the lower end of the scale were content to feed only 6 times in 24 hours, the vast majority required feeding more frequently than this, especially after the first few days.

Observational studies also revealed that the intervals between feeds, for the first few weeks of life at least, were completely random, ranging from 1 to 8 hours.

Subsequently, evidence has accumulated to suggest that babies who are allowed to regulate the frequency of their feeds themselves, gain weight more quickly (26, 27) and remain breastfed for longer (26, 28) than those who have arbitrary rules imposed on them. The evidence provided by such research has formed the basis for the gradual adoption in most maternity units (28) of the more physiological and beneficial practice of demand, or baby-led feeding, which simply consists of feeding the baby whenever he wishes and for as long as he wishes.

Midwives may find, however, that they are caring for breastfeeding women who are still under the mistaken impression that regular, 4-hourly feeding is the normal pattern of behaviour for the majority of breastfed newborn babies. This belief will only serve to undermine confidence in their ability to breastfeed their babies satisfactorily on their breastmilk alone, when they find, as

29

the majority of them will, that their own babies need feeding more frequently than this. A simple explanation of the physiology of lactation and the value of baby-led feeding, both to the baby (reducing the incidence of jaundice (see p. 42) and improving weight gain (26, 27)) and to the mother (in establishing successful lactation (26) and preventing engorgement (see p. 61)) may need to be incorporated tactfully into the early physical assistance that the midwife provides.

Feeding the baby at night
The value of night feeds

Milk production continues as efficiently at night as by day, and if the milk is not removed as it is formed (as regulated by baby's need to go to the breast) the volume of milk in the breast will rapidly exceed the capacity of the alveoli. The consequent engorgement is not only uncomfortable for the mother, but it will begin the process of lactation suppression (29). Feeding the baby at night will minimise or prevent the potential problem of engorgement (see p. 61).

Once lactation is established, night feeds provide the infant with a substantial proportion of his 24-hour intake. The younger the baby, the more likely he is to consume the same volume of milk during the 12 hours from 5pm and 5am as between 5am and 5pm, i.e. 50% on average (30). It is therefore to be expected that the baby will be hungry at night, and assuaging this hunger with formula feeds may lead to lactation suppression in his mother.

Although the long term relationship between prolactin levels and milk production has not been clearly defined (31), it does appear that high levels of prolactin are necessary not only for the initiation of lactation, but are directly related to milk yields in the first 2 weeks at least (32–34). A recent study has demonstrated that prolactin release in response to night time suckling is greater than during the day; thus milk production may get its greatest 'boost' when the baby feeds at night (31, 35).

As prolactin levels have been shown to rise in response to suckling, the practice of baby-led feeding is likely to result in higher basal prolactin levels. The frequent suckling, which results in elevated prolactin levels, also suppresses ovulation, although the exact mechanism is not

30

yet clear (35). The contraceptive effect of breastfeeding, although not 100% reliable, may be of great importance to those who for personal or religious reasons do not wish to use conventional (Western) methods, and it is therefore vital that these women are not subjected to any restrictions on feeds, especially at night.

It is often thought to be a kindness to the newly delivered woman to remove the baby from her bedside so that she can sleep. However the baby will probably sleep for quite a long time after his post-delivery alertness (23, 36). During this time his mother can also sleep if she wishes.

Subsequently the mother needs to be able to put the baby to the breast during the night, not only to stimulate her breasts (37, 38), but to *'practise'* attaching the baby to the breasts while they are still soft, in preparation for effective milk removal. Furthermore a woman delivered in hospital needs to have experienced her baby's feeding patterns 'round the clock' (which is something that women delivered at home will do automatically) so that she does not feel that there are any confidence-sapping gaps in her knowledge when she goes home. This information is especially valuable to primiparous women, given the current practice of shorter hospital stay.

Rooming in

A mother is more likely to sleep soundly in hospital if she has her baby beside her, as she will be confident that if her own baby wakes, she will hear him. She is then less likely to be disturbed by the sound of other babies in the night.

Bedding in

In many cultures the most usual place for a baby to be, night or day, is with his mother (39, 40). Indeed in some societies it would be unsafe for the baby to be anywhere else. In many places the practice is so firmly entrenched that even where women give birth in hospital (e.g. Bombay in India, or Chiang Mai in Thailand) it is expected that the baby will sleep with his mother; some hospitals do not even provide cots (6, 41).

The idea that babies 'should' sleep separately is a fairly recent feature of Western civilisation; in the mid-

31

nineteenth century, Western medical textbooks were still advocating that mother and baby should sleep together, in part to protect the baby from cold (42).

Bedding in has apparently become less common in Western society. Health professionals seem to fear that a baby who shares his mother's bed is at risk, either from falling out of bed or from suffocation. The fears have been greatly exaggerated. Cot deaths, which by comparison are much more common, were in the past thought to be the result of overlaying. There is no evidence, today, to say categorically that bedding in either increases or decreases the incidence of cot death (43).

In the Nair Charitable Hospital in Bombay, for example, where bedding in is common, and has been for many years, there have been no 'accidents' as a result of babies sharing their mother's bed (41). Although the actual number of babies who sleep with their mothers in Britain is unknown, it is undoubtedly more common at home than in hospital.

The most recent OPCS records (1985) show that accidental mechanical suffocation of a baby whilst in its parents' bed is a very rare event. Furthermore the same small number of babies died (in the same year) in their own bed or cradle as died in their parents' bed (44) (see also footnote).

As time-lapse film has demonstrated (45), a healthy baby sleeping with healthy parents moves many times during his periods of sleep, adapting his position to that of his parents, and is usually in no danger of suffocating. It should however be stressed that both baby and parents were well; if either parent were ill, sedated, intoxicated or grossly obese; or if the baby were immobilised in plaster, bedding in might not be advisable. In addition, the type of bedding must be considered, as very soft bedding, or water beds, may increase the risk to the baby (46).

Various solutions are available to those who fear that

FOOTNOTE: OPCS. In 1985 the total number of deaths of babies between birth and one year was 6141. Of these, 6 babies died (in their first year) from accidental mechanical suffocation, 4 in their parents' bed and 2 in their own bed or cradle (a further 1165 died as a result of cot deaths). Figures for 1985 available as: 'Mortality Statistics by Cause'; Annual Ref Vol DH2 1985. HMSO.

the baby may fall out of the bed, despite the presence of his mother. They could both sleep on a mattress on the floor; the bed could have cot-sides attached; it could be pushed up against the wall, or the bedclothes could be firmly tucked around the couple and under the mattress.

Not all mothers wish to sleep with their infants, but there seems to be no reason why those who choose to do so should be dissuaded from following their own inclinations, either in hospital or at home.

Sleep and the mother

Sleep is important to the mother of a young baby, and she may be less disturbed if she uses thicker or more absorbent nappies and does not change the baby at night unless the outer clothes are wet or the baby is fretful. Minimal disturbance of a baby who has wakened only to be fed may result in the baby settling more quickly after the feed. It may also help the baby to begin to appreciate that day and night are different.

The quality of sleep the newly delivered mother experiences may be improved by breastfeeding at night. Although there is no direct experimental evidence to suggest a role for oxytocin in the control of cortical activity (47), there is a suggestion that dopamine receptors in the brain mediate sedation and sleep (48) and that dopamine may be involved in the mechanism of oxytocin release (49). If this is the case, it may account for the often reported and observed (50) sleepiness that many women experience when they breastfeed, which facilitates a rapid return to sleep at night (51).

Monitoring the baby's health and wellbeing

The midwife has responsibilities for the baby, as well as for the mother. This is particularly apparent when the mother and baby go home from hospital and the midwife must monitor the baby's progress for a statutory period. However, not all aspects of the health and wellbeing of a baby can be assessed in relation to a set of standard values. It is not as easy to implement rigid criteria for weight gain, stool frequency and appearance, or the baby's general state of vitality, as it is for serum bilirubin or blood glucose levels.

33

Weight

In the short period after birth for which the midwife attends the mother and baby, it is not possible to establish whether the baby is 'on target' for his genetically determined growth trajectory. The size of the baby at birth, largely determined by placental sufficiency, will not necessarily match this later 'biological size' and there may be a variable period after birth until the balance between these two is reached.

In practice, the simplest and most readily applied 'yardstick' is that the baby should have regained his birth weight by 10 days of age, as an indication that the postnatal physiological losses have been made up. This presupposes that the baby's birth weight was accurately measured and recorded. It should also be borne in mind that there are limitations to the accuracy of midwives' scales (52, 53), and also that the normal daily variability in the baby's weight will make it difficult to establish the baby's absolute weight with any certainty.

It is important to realise that the midwife may influence the mother's expectations about her baby's future growth. If the information that she gives the mother is not soundly based it will create conflict when the mother and baby pass from her care to that of the health visitor.

Weight gain

The appropriateness of applying growth standards derived some years ago from infants who were largely formula fed to the exclusively breastfed baby is currently being questioned (54). Initially, the typical breastfed baby grows rapidly, gaining weight faster than a bottle-fed baby over the first 2–3 months. The rate of gain then slows at around 4 months, ultimately falling below that of the bottle-fed baby at around 6–12 months. Though previously interpreted as 'growth faltering' due to breast milk inadequacy, this pattern is now gaining acceptance as the normal one for a breastfed infant (55).

The actual growth pattern can only be determined by routine monthly weight measurements. Measuring growth reliably over shorter periods (e.g. a week) is much more difficult, particularly so in the first 2 weeks after birth when changes in weight are so dramatic and variable. However, the net gain *over* birth weight in the first fortnight, as estimated from neonatal growth charts (56), is likely to be of the order of 100 g; roughly 20 g per day.

Weight variations

A baby's weight may fluctuate with incidental events such as passing a stool or urine or taking a feed.

In the first few days the infant will pass meconium and lose some water by evaporation. Since the breastfed baby is adapted to taking only small amounts of highly nutritious fluid for the first few days, a net loss of weight would be expected.

It is not possible to abolish day to day variations when monitoring weight, but they can be reduced to a minimum by standardising the times and procedure for measuring weight, e.g. naked weight, before a feed and at the same time of day. If the baby is weighed at set intervals, preferably on the same scales each time, the general trend over time should provide useful information.

However, if conditions are not standardised, or if the baby is weighed too frequently, incidental changes such as a breastfeed (of, say 150 g) or the passage of a stool and urine (say, 180 g) will entirely swamp the anticipated daily weight increment cited earlier, i.e. 20 g/day.

Although it would be appropriate for the midwife to be concerned if a baby was gaining weight more slowly than expected, she should be aware that expressing too much anxiety in the mother's presence may be counter-productive. It may have the effect of damaging the mother's confidence in her ability to breastfeed, which may in itself be detrimental to her milk supply.

The issue of whether the infant subsequently showed a satisfactory weight gain would have to be considered in relation to other factors, such as parental stature or gestational age, in order to assess the anticipated growth pattern of the infant in question.

Stools

The passage of the first stool by the newborn is usually indicative of a patent intestinal tract, and this fact is noted in most hospital and community settings today. The length of time taken for meconium to change to the yellow stool of the milk-fed neonate will vary according to gestational age, feeding methods and patterns, and can give some

35

indication of the baby's wellbeing in relation to his milk intake.

Initially the stools of a breastfed baby will vary in number and amount, and will depend on the intake of colostrum. Breastmilk, a complete food, is fully utilised, and the baby's stools may appear quite loose on or around the 3rd day of life. This corresponds with the mother's milk 'coming in' and is quite normal. Thereafter the mother should be advised that her baby will continue to have quite loose stools for as long as he remains exclusively breastfed.

Breastfed babies' bowels do not necessarily move at regular intervals, and provided that the baby is well there should be no cause for concern. No intervention is necessary and the baby is not constipated as is often suggested. It is unnecessary and unacceptable to give a breastfed baby sugary drinks (see pp. 41–44).

The following is offered as a guide to the stool colour change expected in a healthy term infant:-

Birth–24 hours	=	1st day meconium
24–48 hours	=	2nd day meconium/changing
48–72 hours	=	3rd day changing/yellow
72–96 hours	=	4th day yellow

A term baby, who is still passing meconium at 4–5 days is probably getting insufficient milk for his needs and losing weight. Similarly, stools described as 'changing' at 4–5 days could indicate some shortcoming in relation to breastfeeding procedure, e.g. incorrect positioning or restricting the duration or the frequency of feeds.

General health

Weight gain is only one of a number of indications that the newborn infant is healthy, and thriving on his mother's milk. The stature of parents, while not wholly reliable, is the 'best' indication of the future size of the infant. Thus if the infant does not appear to be gaining weight, but in all other respects seems to be happy and healthy, there should be no immediate cause for concern.

Other vital signs include:

1. Good skin colour; not grey or pale.
2. Alert and responsive.

3. Frequent 'wet' nappies with pale, odourless urine. (This sign is only useful if the infant is being exclusively breastfed, i.e. no supplementary or complementary feeds.)

4. Normal stools for age – see above.

5. Contented most of the time (i.e. not constantly fretful or crying) but without being lethargic.

Just as these can be considered positive signs in a baby who is not gaining weight, so too, if there is adequate weight gain but there are clear deficits in any of the above, there should be cause for concern.

References

Advice and support at the first feed

1. De Chateau P 1980 The First Hour After Delivery. Its Impact on Synchrony of Parent–Infant Relationship. Paediatrician 9: 151–168
2. Salariya EM, Easton PM, Cater Jl 1978 Duration of Feeding After Early Initiation and Frequent Feeding. Lancet ii 1141–1143
3. Winters NW 1973 The Relationship of Time of Initial Breastfeeding to Success in Breastfeeding. Unpublished Master's Thesis, University of Washington.
   See also:
   Johnson NW (same author) 1986 Breastfeeding at One Hour of Age. American Journal of Maternal and Child Nursing Jan/Feb pp 12–16
4. De Chateau P, Wiberg B 1977 Long Term Effect on Mother–Infant Behaviour of Extra Contact During the First Hour Post-Partum. Acta Paediatrica Scandinavica 66: 137–151
5. Thomsen MF, Hartstock TG, Larson C 1979 The Importance of Immediate Post-Natal Contact: Its Effects on Breastfeeding. Canadian Family Physician 25: 1374–1378
6. Woolridge MW, Greasley V, Silpisolnosol S 1985 The Initiation of Lactation: Effect of Early Delayed Contact for Suckling on Milk Intake in the First Week Post-Partum. A study in Chang Mai, Northern Thailand. Early Human Development 12: 269–278
7. Widstrom AM, Ransjo-Arvidson AB, Christensson K, Mattiesen AS, Winberg J, Vvnas-Moberg K 1987 Gastric Suction in Healthy Newborn Infants. Acta Paediatrica Scandinavica 76: 566–572
8. Garforth S, Garcia J In: Inch S 1987 Difficulties With Breastfeeding – Midwives in Disarray? Journal of the Royal Society of Medicine 80: 53–57
9. Gunther M 1955 Instinct and the Nursing Couple. Lancet i: 575–578

Unrestricted feeds

10. King FT 1913 Feeding and Care of the Baby. Macmillan, London
11. Naish L 1913 Breastfeeding – Its Management and Mismanagement. Lancet i: pp 1657–1659
12. Liddiard M 1924–48 The Mothercraft Manual. J & A Churchill, London

37

Factors which have been shown to help

4

13. Slaven S, Harvey D 1981 Unlimited Sucking Time Improves Breastfeeding. Lancet i: pp 392–393
14. Carvahlo M et al 1984 Does the Duration and Frequency of Early Breastfeeding Affect Nipple Pain? Vol 11: 2 (Summer): 81–84
15. Kries RV et al 1987 Vitamin K_1 Content of Maternal Milk: Influence of the Stage of Lactation, Lipid Composition and Vitamin K_1 Supplements given to the Mother. Paediatric Research Vol 22 No 5
16. Woolridge M, Fisher C 1988 Colic, 'Overfeeding' and Symptoms of Malabsorption in the Breast-fed Baby: A Possible Artefact of Feed Management? Lancet ii: 382–384
17. Hytten F 1954 Clinical Studies in Lactation 11: Variation in the Major Constituents During a Feeding. British Medical Journal 1: 176–179.
18. Hall B 1975 Changing Composition of Milk and Early Development of an Appetite Control. Lancet i: 779–781
19. Woolridge MW et al 1982 Individual Patterns of Milk Intake During Breastfeeding. Early Human Development 7: 265–272
20. Lucas A et al 1979 Patterns of Milk Flow in Breastfed Babies. Lancet ii (8133): 57–58
21. Fisher C In: Inch S 1987 Difficulties with Breastfeeding – Midwives in Disarray? Journal of the Royal Society of Medicine 80: 53–54
22. Simsarian FP, McLendon PA 1942 Feeding Behaviour of an Infant During the First Twelve Weeks of Life on a Self-demand Schedule. Journal of Paediatrics 20: 93–103
23. Simsarian FP, McLendon PA 1945 Further Records of the Self-demand Schedule in Infant-Feeding. Journal of Paediatrics 17: 109–114
24. Olmsted RW, Jackson EB 1950 Self-demand Feeding in the First Week of Life. Paediatrics 6: 396–401
25. Carvahlo M et al 1982 Effect of Frequent Breastfeeding on Early Milk Production and Infant Weight Gain. Paediatrics 72 (3): 307–311
26. Illingworth RS, Stone DG 1952 Self-demand Feeding in a Maternity Unit. Lancet i: 683–687
27. Salver EJ 1956 The Effect of Different Feeding Schedules on the Growth of Bantu Babies in the First Week of Life. Journal of Tropical Paediatrics September: 97–102
28. Martin J, Monk M 1982 Infant Feeding 1980. Office of Population Census and Surveys. Social Survey Division. pp 40–44

Feeding the baby at night
29. Dawson EK 1935 Edinburgh Medical Journal 42: 569
30. Dewey KG, Lonnerdal B 1983 Breast Milk Intake: Variations in Feeding Practices. American Journal of Clinical Nutrition July: 152–153 (letter)
31. Glasier AS, McNeilly AS, Howie PW 1984 The Prolactin Response to Suckling. Clinical Endocrinology 21: 109–116
32. Aono T, Aki T, Koike K, Kurachi K 1982 Effects of Sulpiride on

Poor Lactation. American Journal of Obstetrics and Gynecology 143: 927–932

33. Kauppila A, Kivinen S, Ylikorkala O 1981 Metoclopramide Increases Prolactin Release and Milk Secretion in the Puerperium Without Stimulating the Secretion of Thyrotropin and Thyroid Hormones. Journal of Clinical Endocrinology and Metabolism 52: 436–439

34. Ylikorkala O, Kauppila A, Kivinen S, Vinikka L 1982 Sulpiride Improves Inadequate Lactation. British Medical Journal 285: 249–250

35. Howie PW 1985 Breastfeeding – A New Understanding. Midwives Chronicle and Nursing Notes July: 184–192

36. Macfarlane A 1977 The Psychology of Childbirth. Fontana Open Books, London, p 76

37. Krnjevic K, Phillis JW, 1963 Pharmacological Properties of ACh Sensitive Cells in the Cerebral Cortex. Journal of Physiology 166: 328–350

38. McNeilly AS, Robinson IC, Houston MJ, Howie PW 1983 Release of Prolactin and Oxytocin in Response to Suckling. British Medical Journal 287: 257–259

39. Mead M 1976 Quoted on the back cover of: Thevenin T The Family Bed. Published by Thevenin, PO Box 16004, Minneapolis, MN 55416, USA

40. Liedloff J 1975 The Continuum Concept. Futura Publications, p 46

41. Anand RK 1981 The Management of Breastfeeding in a Bombay Hospital. In: Assignment Children 2. 55–56 Breastfeeding and Health. UNICEF, p 172

42. Coombe A 1840 Management of Infancy, NY Fowlers and Wells 207, quoted in The Family Bed. Thevenin, Minneapolis, USA

43. Personal Communication (Reed J) 1987 The Foundation for the Study of Infant Deaths. 15 Belgrave Square, London SW1 8PS

44. OCPS Figures for 1985, Mortality Statistics by Cause. Annual Reference Volume DH2 1985. HMSO, London

45. Julian Aston Productions 1978 Newman Pass, London W1. First shown on Tomorrow's World

46. Bass M, Kravath RE, Glass L 1986 Death Scene Investigation in Sudden Infant Death. New England Journal of Medicine 315 (2): 100 105

47. Paisley AC, Summerlee AJS 1984 Relationships Between Behavioural States and Activity in the Cerebral Cortex. Progress in Neurobiology 22 (2): 155–184

48. Corsini GU 1977 Evidence for Dopamine Receptors in the Human Brain Mediating Sedation and Sleep. Life Sciences 20(a): 1613–1618

49. Clark G, Lincoln DW, Merrick I, 1979 Dopaminergic Control of Oxytocin Release in Lactating Rats. Journal of Endocrinology 83: 409–420

50. Bourne MA 1983 Sleep and the Newborn. New Generation 2 (2): 16–17

51. Urnas-Moberg K 1989 The Gastrointestinal Tract in Growth and Reproduction. Scientific American July: 60–65

Factors which have been shown to help

Monitoring infant health and wellbeing

52. Culley P, Milan P, Roginski C, Waterhouse J, Wood B 1979 Are Breastfed Babies Still Getting a Raw Deal in Hospital? British Medical Journal ii: 891–893
53. Whitfield MF, Kay R, Stevens S 1981 Validity of Routine Clinical Test Weighing as a Measure of the Intake of Breastfed Infants. Archives of Diseases in Childhood 56: 919–921
54. Whitehead RG, Paul AA 1985 Growth Charts and the Assessment of Infant Feeding Practices in the Western World and in Developing Countries. Early Human Development 9: 187–207
55. Wood CS, Isaacs PC, Jensen M, Hilton HG 1988 Exclusively Breastfed Infants: Growth and Calorie Intake. Pediatric Nursing March/April Vol 14 No 2
56. Gardner D, Pearson J 1971 A Growth Chart for Premature and Other Infants. Archives of Diseases in Childhood 46: 783–787

Factors which have been shown to be unhelpful

Additional fluids for breastfed babies 41
Test weighing 44
Maternal dietary modifications 45

Additional fluids for breastfed babies

Supplementary and complementary feeds – of either water, glucose/dextrose or formula have not been shown in any of the trials reviewed below (or in any of the randomised controlled trials in the Oxford Database of perinatal trials) to be of any benefit to healthy, term, breastfed infants.

Midwives should remember that bottle-feeding does not resolve breastfeeding problems but knowledgeable, enthusiastic and sympathetic help can.

Dehydration

The volume of colostrum/milk available to the newborn infant increases rapidly in the first 3 days after birth from a range of 7 to 122.5 ml/24 hours (1) and a mean of 7.5 ml/feed in the first 24 hours after birth; to a range of 98 to 775 ml/24 hours and a mean of 38 ml/feed by the 3rd postnatal day (2). There is no evidence to suggest that a healthy term baby has a need for large volumes of fluid any earlier than they are made available physiologically.

To date at least two trials have been undertaken to examine the suggestion that healthy babies, who are exclusively breastfed, need extra water in hot weather. The studies measured the urine concentration of the babies, found that it was well within the normal range and concluded that no additional water was necessary, even in hot weather (3, 4).

Jaundice

Various researchers have investigated the seemingly widespread belief that giving additional fluids to a breastfed baby prevents or resolves physiological jaundice. Nicoll et al (5) randomly allocated 49 breastfed babies to three groups: no supplement, water supplement and dextrose supplement. Despite the observation that the infants in the dextrose group consumed a significantly greater mean volume of fluid than those in the water group, those in the no supplement group had the lowest mean serum bilirubin levels on the 6th day.

Carvahlo et al (6) compared two groups of breastfed babies, one of which received supplementary water and one of which did not, and Herrera (7) similarly compared two groups, one of which received supplementary glucose while the other did not. They found no difference in the number of babies who developed jaundice, the number who required phototherapy or in the mean serum bilirubin, between the two groups.

Kuhr and Paneth (8) recorded the total amount of supplementary dextrose given over a 72 hour period to 77 consecutively born, healthy, term, breastfed babies, test weighed them on the 4th day and analysed the results in relation to those who appeared jaundiced and thus had their serum bilirubin levels measured. They found babies who took large volumes of dextrose supplement in the first 3 days of life not only tended to take less milk per feed by the 4th day, but were also more likely to be jaundiced than those who did not. None of the researchers found any relationship between the degree of weight loss and the development of physiological jaundice (5–7, 9).

On the basis of the evidence, the most effective way of reducing the incidence of physiological jaundice in breastfed babies would appear to be to ensure that no limitations are placed on the frequency with which the babies go to their mother's breast.

Hazards of additional fluids

The fact that a practice cannot be shown to be of benefit ought to be sufficient reason for abandoning it, especially in the present economic climate. In 1980 it was estimated that a hospital which delivered 5000 babies per year, of whom 70% were initially breastfed, was paying out £7000 per year on prepacked supplementary feeds of water and dextrose! (5).

More important still are the observations that supplementary fluids may ultimately reduce the length of time for which a mother breastfeeds her baby; either by undermining her confidence, or by impairing her ability to establish effective lactation. The mechanism by which artificial feeding undermines the mother's attempts to breastfeed may be partly psychological, in that she becomes accustomed to seeing and measuring the quantity of milk taken by the baby.

This of course is not necessary for successful breastfeeding but the mother may doubt her ability to produce quantities of milk because she does not see it.

De Chateau et al (10) compared two groups of breastfeeding women, one for whom test weighing and supplementation were routine, with one for whom this practice was discontinued. They found that five times as many mothers stopped breastfeeding in the first week in the supplemented group, and twice as many stopped in the second week.

A year later, when the practice had been discontinued through the unit, they found that the mean duration of breastfeeding was 95 days, compared with the former 42 days.

Bergevin et al (11) randomly allocated a large number of breastfeeding women into two groups; one group received a sample of formula when they left the hospital and the other did not. They found that even this small intervention was sufficient to increase the number of women who had stopped breastfeeding at 1 month, and who had introduced solids by 2 months.

The difference between the two groups was even greater in 'vulnerable' groups, such as primiparae, the less well educated and those who became ill postnatally. Yet in many hospitals prepacked feeds of even water and glucose bear the name of a manufacturer of infant formula which in itself can act as a form of advertising (12).

Both Herrera (7) and Gray Donald et al (13) found significantly fewer women who were still breastfeeding at

43

4, 9 and 12 weeks after the birth of their babies, if their babies had received supplementary fluids in hospital, compared with those whose babies had been exclusively breastfed. This may, in turn, have repercussions on the future health of genetically susceptible infants (14).

Although this remains controversial, the wishes of the parents should be respected. Many researchers have shown the value of exclusive breastfeeding to the children of parents with allergies (15–17).

Both cow's milk-based formula and soya-based formula are potential allergens, and may play a role in the aetiology of conditions such as eczema and asthma.

Parents suffering from these conditions deserve every help in their attempts to avoid sensitising their children (18). If supplementation is essential for some reason, human milk will be less risky for such infants.

Test weighing

Under normal circumstances test weighing is neither a necessary nor an effective tool for assessing the adequacy of lactation.

Test weighing is normally understood to mean calculating the amount of breastmilk consumed at a feed by weighing the baby before and after that feed and subtracting the first weighing from the second.

Modern electronic scales are now available for weighing babies. The older type of mechanical scales have neither sufficient precision nor the accuracy necessary for measuring small intakes of breastmilk. Their use can lead to errors of + or –30 g, which may be as large as the intake being measured (19–21).

It may also be positively harmful to a mother's confidence in her ability to breastfeed if a single test weighing appears to show that the baby has consumed what may be regarded as an inadequate volume.

The measurement of only one feed may be unrepresentative of other feeds taken throughout the day, particularly if the test weigh is carried out under conditions which are perceived as threatening to the mother, as this may impair milk transfer.

Measuring only volume intake, without a knowledge of the calorie content of the milk consumed, may give a misleading picture of the nutritional adequacy of the baby's diet.

If it is necessary to know how much milk a breastfed baby is consuming, test weighing should be carried out over a complete 24 hour period, using an electronic, averaging scale (or a heavily 'damped' electronic scale) in order to establish the volume intake accurately.

Maternal dietary modifications

The advice given to breastfeeding women concerning their optimum food and drink intake has long been the subject of debate, and in this area, as in so many others, much of the advice has been conflicting.

Additional fluids for breastfeeding mothers

Over 30 years ago researchers demonstrated that a baby's weight was not significantly improved by deliberately increasing the mother's fluid intake (22). More recently, other studies have shown that neither a significant decrease, (23) nor a significant increase (23, 24) in maternal fluid intake has any effect on milk production.

Thus thirst will effectively regulate the fluid intake of a lactating woman, just as it does with all other lactating mammals; and the practice of encouraging breastfeeding women to drink large quantities of liquid should be abandoned.

They might, however, be reminded that dark, strongly smelling urine is an indication that they need to drink more.

Additional calories for breastfeeding mothers

It has become apparent over the past few years that the theoretical calculation of the number of extra calories that a lactating woman needs to obtain from her diet is not borne out in practice. This calculation was based on an assumption that to provide 800 ml of milk (560 cals) she would have to make some 700 calories available for milk production (the efficiency of milk production being about 80% (25)).

Recent dietary surveys in developed countries performed on well nourished women with healthy babies have consistently found their calorie intake to be less than the recommended amount (26, 27). Furthermore, controlled trials conducted in developing countries have demonstrated that giving extra food to mothers, even those who were poorly nourished, did not increase the rate of growth of their babies (28–32).

A possible explanation for these findings has been supplied by Illingworth et al (33), who found that metabolic efficiency was enhanced in lactating women, who were therefore able to conserve energy and 'subsidise' the cost of their milk production.

Thus hunger will effectively regulate the calorie intake of a breastfeeding woman, just as it does in all other lactating mammals, and the practice of encouraging breastfeeding mothers to eat excessively should be abandoned. They might, however, need advice regarding the nature of a 'well balanced diet' which is so often recommended without further explanation.

Dietary prohibitions for breastfeeding mothers

As a general rule, there is no reason to advise a lactating woman that she should omit any particular food from her diet, just because she is breastfeeding. Any food may be consumed in moderation, unless or until the situation dictates otherwise. However, a woman with a family history of allergy may benefit from some modification of her diet, during both pregnancy and lactation (18).

She should be reassured that the very loose stools that her baby may have from the 3rd to the 5th day of life are a perfectly normal response to the influx of milk which occurs at this time, and are unlikely to be related to maternal dietary indiscretions.

However, it appears that there are some foods which may have an allergenic effect on particular babies when ingested by their mothers (18, 34). If there is any reason to suspect that any food the mother has eaten has been responsible for some adverse reaction in the baby, the mother should avoid that food for 2 weeks and then return to it. If the baby's condition deteriorates again, the mother should avoid the food completely and seek additional dietary advice (35).

Provision of free samples to mothers

Giving infant formula to breastfed babies in their 1st week of life has been found to be the most important variable predicting the cessation of breastfeeding in the first 2 weeks (36). It has also been shown that giving samples of formula to breastfeeding mothers is likely to shorten the period for which they breastfeed, as well as encouraging the early introduction of solid food (37). Lactational failure in this context is a result of the combined effects of lack of confidence and reduced suckling (38). Giving free samples to mothers can also imply recommendation of a brand, and thus becomes an effective way of promoting brand sales (39). It also raises doubts in the mother's mind about the degree to which those caring for her are committed to breastfeeding. There is no reason why breastfeeding mothers of healthy, term infants should be given samples of ready-to-feed formula, water or glucose, even in hospital. They should not be given to any mother on discharge from hospital and particularly not to breastfeeding mothers.

In the UK, women who wish to bottle-feed and who are receiving Income Support or Family Credit are entitled to milk tokens, which can be exchanged for two (450 g) packets of infant formula per week. This should be adequate for any baby who is bottle-fed, and it should not be necessary for the mother to be given free samples by the hospital when she goes home.

Promotion of breastmilk substitutes

As a result of international collaboration between the World Health Organization (WHO), the United Nations International Children's Emergency Fund (UNICEF), medical experts, government representatives, infant food industry personnel and the consumer groups, a voluntary Code for the Marketing of Breastmilk Substitutes has been developed (40). The Code seeks to contribute to safe, adequate nutrition for infants, promote and protect breastfeeding, ensure the correct use of breastmilk substitutes and control the use of questionable marketing techniques in the selling of products for bottle-feeding.

47

Factors which have been shown to be unhelpful

5

The Code does not prevent mothers from bottle-feeding if that is what they choose to do. The object of the Code is to control unethical marketing to parents and staff in health care facilities, and to reduce the pressure that some companies exert on health professionals. It seeks to encourage and maintain the woman's right to breastfeed, and the baby's right to have access to his mother's own milk. Nowhere does it seek to enforce breastfeeding. The Code applies to all breastmilk substitutes for babies; including follow-on milks and other products which can be given using a feeding bottle, as well as utensils used for bottle-feeding, such as feeding bottles and teats. Included in the Articles of the Code are:

1. No advertising of these products to the public.
2. No free samples to mothers or members of their families.
3. No promotion of products in health care facilities.
4. No company personnel to advise mothers or members of their families.
5. No gifts or personal samples to health workers.
6. No words or pictures idealising bottle-feeding, including pictures of infants on the labels of the products.
7. All information on infant feeding, including product labels, should explain the benefits of breastfeeding and the costs and hazards associated with bottle-feeding.
8. Unsuitable products, such as sweetened condensed milk should not be promoted for babies.
9. All products should be of high quality, and should take into account the climatic and storage conditions of the country where they are to be used.

The Code recommends that health care facilities and staff should not be used for the purposes of advertising and promoting bottle-feeding to the public: this recommendation includes the display of calendars and posters, as well as the use of cot tags, tape measures, leaflets, baby booklets and mugs.

At the 1981 World Health Assembly, Britain voted in favour of the WHO Code. It is an International Code and therefore applies worldwide. It was set down as a minimum requirement to protect infant health, and it is the responsibility of national governments to formulate their

48

Codes based on the WHO Code. Britain has its own Code known as the Food Manufacturers Federation Code (FMF Code (41)), but this falls short of the WHO Code (40) in many important areas. It only applies to the direct advertising of infant formulae. Other products such as infant teas and follow-on milks are not included in the scope of the FMF code. An up-dated circular from the Department of Health HC(89)21 (42) makes firm recommendations to health service staff; that they should neither accept nor distribute free samples of infant formula, and Health Authorities should refuse subsidised supplies of infant formulae. However, advertising is still permitted within the Health Service since commercial handbooks and leaflets on feeding for mothers, according to Health Circular HC(89)21 (42), can contain advertising for infant formulae. It is easy to understand why mothers may gain the impression that bottle-feeding is equivalent to breastfeeding if the health care facility endorses such practices.

There is now also a Code of Marketing of infant bottles and teats as an annexe, which is closely modelled on the FMF code. The FMF Code may have to be revised if the EEC legislates to adopt the WHO Code for its member states.

Any individual, professional or private, who perceives a breach of the FMF guidelines, can complain to the Code Monitoring Committee, which is in turn required to report to the Secretaries of State on the functioning of the FMF Code (42). Midwives wishing to report violations of the stricter WHO Code can send details to consumer organisations urging the adoption of the WHO Code for Britain.

References

Additional fluids for breastfed babies

1. Saint L et al 1984 The Yield and Nutrient Content of Colostrum and Milk of Women from Giving Birth to One Month Post Partum. British Journal of Nutrition 52: 87–95
2. Houston MJ et al 1983 Factors Affecting the Duration of Breastfeeding: 1. Measurement of Breast Milk Intake in the First Week of Life. Early Human Development 8: 49–54
3. Almroth SG 1978 Water Requirements of Breastfed Babies in a Hot Climate. American Journal of Clinical Nutrition 31: 1154–1157
4. Goldberg NM, Adams E 1983 Supplementary Water for Breastfed

Factors which have been shown to be unhelpful

Babies in a Hot Dry Climate – Not Really a Necessity. Achives of Diseases in Childhood January: 73–74

5. Nicoll A et al 1982 Supplementary Feeding and Jaundice in Newborns. Acta Paediatrica Scandinavica 71: 759–761

6. Carvahlo M et al 1981 Effect of Water Supplementation on Physiological Jaundice in Breastfed Babies. Archives of Diseases in Childhood 56 (7): 568–569

7. Herrera AJ 1984 Supplemented Versus Unsupplemented Breastfeeding. Perinatology – Neonatology 8 (3): 70–71

8. Kuhr M, Paneth N 1982 Feeding Practices and Early Neonatal Jaundice. Journal of Paediatrics, Gastroenterology and Nutrition 1: 485–488

9. Carvahlo M et al 1982 Frequency of Breastfeeding and Serum Bilirubin Concentration. American Journal of Diseases of Children 136: 737–738

10. De Chateau P et al 1977 A Study of Factors Promoting and Inhibiting Lactation. Developmental Medicine and Child Neurology 19: 575–584

11. Bergevin Y, Dougherty C, Kramer MS 1983 Do Infant Formula Samples Shorten the Duration of Breastfeeding? Lancet i: 1148–1151

12. Lobstein T 1987 Warding off the Bottle. The London Food Commission.

13. Gray-Donald K et al 1985 Effect of Formula Supplementation in Hospital on the Duration of Breastfeeding: A Controlled Trial. Paediatrics 75 (3): 514–518

14. Borch-Johnsen K et al 1984 Relation Between Breastfeeding and Incidence Rates of Insulin Dependent Diabetes Mellitus. Lancet ii: 1083–1086

15. Minchin M 1985 Breastfeeding Matters. Allen & Unwin, Australia and 1985 Food for Thought – A Parent's Guide to Food Intolerance. Oxford University Press, Oxford.

16. Jelliffe DD, Jelliffe EFP 1978 Human Milk in the Modern World. Oxford University Press, London.

17. Evensen S 1983 Relationship Between Infant Morbidity and Breastfeeding Versus Artificial Feeding in Industrialized Countries: A Review of the Literature. Issued by the World Health Organization Regional Office for Europe. ICP NUT 010/6 Rev. 1 0292M. Obtainable by Mail Order from: HMSO Publications Centre, 51 Nine Elms Lane, London SW8 5DR

18. Chandra RK, Puri S, Suraika C et al 1986 Influence of Maternal Food Avoidance During Pregnancy and Lactation on the Incidence of Atopic Eczema in Infants. Clinical Allergy 16: 563–569

Test Weighing

19. Culley P, Milan P, Roginski C, Waterhouse J, Wood B 1979 Are Breastfed Babies Still Getting a Raw Deal in Hospital? British Medical Journal 2: 891–893

20. Whitfield MF, Kay R, Stevens S 1981 Validity of Routine Test Weighing as a Measure of the Intake of Breastfed Infants. Archives of Diseases in Childhood 56: 919–921

21. Drewett RF, Woolridge MW, Greasley V et al 1984 Evaluating Breastmilk Intake by Test Weighing: A Portable Electronic Balance Suitable for Community and Field Studies. Early Human Development 10: 123–126

Maternal dietary modifications

22. Illingworth RS, Kilpatrick B 1953 Lactation and Fluid Intake. Lancet ii: 1175–1177
23. Dearlove JC, Dearlove BM 1981 Prolactin, Fluid Balance and Lactation. British Journal of Obstetrics and Gynaecology 123: 845–846
24. Dusdicker LB et al 1985 Effect of Supplementary Fluids on Human Milk Production. Journal of Paediatrics 106: 207–211
25. National Research Council. 1980 Recommended Dietary Allowances. 9th edn. Washington National Academy of Sciences.
26. Whitehead RG, Paul AA, Black AE, Wiles SJ 1981 Recommended Dietary Amounts of Energy for Pregnancy or Lactation in the UK. In: Torun B, Young VR, Rang WM (eds) Protein Energy Requirements of Developing Countries: Evaluation of New Data. United Nations University, Tokyo: 259–265
27. Butte NF, Garza C, Stuff JE, Smith EO, Bichos BJ 1984 Effect of Maternal Diet and Body Composition on Lactational Performance. American Journal of Clinical Nutrition 39: 296–306
28. Blackwell RQ, Chow BF, Chinn KSK, Blackwell BN 1973 Prospective Maternal Nutrition Study in Taiwan: Rationale, Study Design Feasibility and Preliminary Findings. Nutrition Reports International 7: 517–532
29. Delgado HL, Marmtorell R, Klein RE 1982 Nutrition, Lactation and Birth Interval Components In Rural Guatemala. American Journal of Clinical Nutrition 35: 1468–1476
30. Prentice AM, Roberts SB, Whitehead RG 1980 Dietary Supplementation of Gambian Nursing Mothers and Lactational Performance. Lancet ii: 886–888
31. Prentice AM, Whitehead RG, Roberts SB 1983 Dietary Supplementation of Lactating Gambian Women. I. Effect on Breastmilk Volume and Quality. Human Nutrition and Clinical Nutrition 37(c): 53–64
32. Prentice AM, Lunn PG, Watkinson M, Whitehead RG 1983 Dietary Supplementation of Lactating Gambian Women. II. Effect on Maternal Health, Nutritional Status and Biochemistry. Human Nutrition and Clinical Nutrition 37(c): 65–74
33. Illingworth PJ, Jong RT, Howie PW, Leslie P, Isles TE 1986 Diminution in Energy Expenditure During Lactation. British Medical Journal 292: 437–441
34. Gerrard JW 1980 Adverse Reactions to Foods in Breastfed Babies. In: Freier S, Eidelman A (eds) Human Milk – Its Biological and Social Value. Selected papers from the International Symposium on Breastfeeding. Tel Aviv, pp 170–175
35. Cant AJ, Bailes JA, Marsden RA, Hewitt D 1986 Effect of Maternal Dietary Exclusion on Breastfed Infants with Eczema: Two Controlled Studies. British Medical Journal 293: 231–233

51

Factors which have been shown to be unhelpful

Provision of free samples to mothers

36. Martin J Monk J 1980 Infant Feeding. Social Survey Division, OPCS, London
37. Bergevin Y, Dougherty C, Kramer MS 1983 Do Infant Formula Samples Shorten Breastfeeding? Lancet i: 1148–1151
38. Houston MJ, Howie PW 1981 The Importance of Support for the Breastfeeding Mother. Health Visitor 54 (6): 243
39. Hamilton R, Whinnett D 1986 A comparison of the WHO and United Kingdom Codes of Practice for Marketing of Breastmilk Substitutes. University of Lancaster

Promotion of breastmilk substitutes

40. WHO 1981 International Code of Marketing of Breastmilk Substitutes. World Health Organization, Geneva
41. FMF Code 1983 Available from The Food and Drink Federation, 6 Catherine Street, London WC2
42. Health Circular HC (89) 21 Available from DHSS Store, Health Publications Unit, No 2 Site, Manchester Road, Heywood, Lancashire OL10 2PZ

Successful breastfeeding

Antenatal and postnatal considerations

Influencing the decision to breastfeed 53
Sustaining the decision to breastfeed 54
Prevention of feeding problems 56
Postnatal care of the breasts 57
Treatment of sore nipples 58
Prevention and treatment of engorgement 60
Prevention and treatment of mastitis 62

Influencing the decision to breastfeed

In this society, the majority of women who decide to breastfeed seem to make this decision prior to, or very early in pregnancy (1, 2). Those who choose to bottle feed tend to make up their minds later in pregnancy (1).

Giving well designed, written and illustrated information about breastfeeding to women has been shown to increase (or reinforce) their knowledge of the subject, but it is unlikely to affect their choice of feeding method, or increase the duration of breastfeeding (3). It is more likely that their choice will be affected by socially acquired attitudes and the support that they feel they will get from their families and friends (2, 4). Persuasive campaigns in the mass media and in clinics have been found to have little effect on feeding practices (5–7). Furthermore, once a woman has decided how she will feed her baby, she is unlikely to change her mind (3), although the impact of information indicating that bottle-feeding is problematic has not yet been tested.

As can be seen from pages 56–58, no form of antenatal preparation of the breasts has been shown to be of benefit; thus asking a woman in early pregnancy how she plans to feed her baby is not only unnecessary, it may even be counter-productive if she has not already decided to breastfeed and feels pressured into making a decision. If, in the course of the discussion between mother and midwife, it becomes apparent that the mother would like more information, then it should be provided, otherwise it could be safely left until the last trimester of pregnancy.

Midwives who feel strongly that 'breast is best' have a difficult task in giving information to women who are

53

undecided about their feeding method, or who have chosen to bottle-feed. At no stage should the mother be given the impression that bottle-feeding is equivalent to breastfeeding, or without risk. In particular, women with a strong family history of allergy should be informed that their decision to breastfeed may prevent serious illness in their children. However, there is a subtle but important difference between the heavy-handed approach which makes mothers feel guilty, and the more sensitive approach which allows mothers to make their own decision.

Antenatal classes

One study has demonstrated that one antenatal breastfeeding class, given in the last 2 months of pregnancy to women who have already decided to breastfeed, had a significant positive effect, not only on the duration of breastfeeding but on the way in which the mother perceived herself and her baby postnatally (8). This class (given by an enthusiastic midwife) contained information on the anatomy and physiology of lactation (see pp. 1–6), how to breastfeed (see pp. 13–20), self-care of the breastfeeding mother, possible set-backs early in breastfeeding and their treatments (see pp. 58–59) breastfeeding and the working mother, and resources for the breastfeeding mother (how to get help from both professional and voluntary organisations).

Sustaining the decision to breastfeed

In addition to factors already mentioned, such as early contact and early suckling, other aspects of postnatal care have also been shown to increase the length of time for which a woman breastfeeds.

In one study, a group of women who were given a short, personal, bedside teaching session, while still in hospital, were compared with two others; one group just received a card with the name and phone number of a professional feeding advisor, and the other group were given the same card, plus a manual containing the sort of information that had been given at the teaching session.

Significantly more women who had received the individual tuition were still breastfeeding at 1 month postpartum, compared with the other two groups (9). The effectiveness of this personal, professional contact should encourage midwives to give this aspect of their role high priority.

Another study identified the baby and the baby's father as the greatest sources of encouragement to the mother's breastfeeding attempts; and the woman's own mother as the greatest source of discouragement if she herself had not breastfed (1). The findings of both of these studies could be utilised if the personal, professional helping session was given at the first feed, in the peace and quiet after the newly delivered mother and baby had been attended to and made clean and comfortable, and while the father was still present.

The baby's behaviour and needs can be explained to the usually highly receptive parents, so that in future the baby will not be regarded as being in any way critical or manipulative. The mother's breast and nipple can be considered in relation to the baby's mouth, head and body; the importance of correct positioning and the concept of supply and demand briefly explained (10). (For further details of the first teaching session, see pp. 25–27.)

The other factor that has been shown to be of benefit is prolonged, intermittent postnatal contact with the mother (11). Despite the fact that the study in question was not designed to promote breastfeeding by means of this intervention, but to find why women stopped breastfeeding, the researchers found that more women in the group who were telephoned weekly (in order to be interviewed) throughout the period of breastfeeding, were still breastfeeding at 6 months, when compared to a control group who were interviewed retrospectively. If the interviewer discovered that the woman being telephoned had a problem, it was possible to offer immediate, competent, practical help. This is a role that the voluntary breastfeeding organisations could effectively undertake (perhaps in some modified form), if contact could be made with the mother in the early postnatal period. One of the advantages of extending midwifery care to 28 days is that the mother receives prolonged, intermittent contact, as well as more consistent advice. With good inter-professional communication these advantages should continue when the care of the mother and baby pass to the health visitor.

Prevention of feeding problems

Breastfeeding is a normal physiological process – a natural consequence of giving birth, and in many countries is still the only reliable means of ensuring the survival and healthy growth of a newborn baby.

Breastfeeding problems are likely only when the physiological process is impeded, either by surrounding it with man-made rules and regulations, or by failing to attach the baby to the breast correctly (see pp. 3–6).

However, where this has not been understood, an explanation that is frequently given for the prevalence of breastfeeding problems in Western cultures – despite the lack of evidence to support it – is that they are due to the thinness or sensitivity of the nipple skin. This misconception has unfortunately formed the basis of most of the advice given, and breast preparation advocated, in the antenatal and postnatal period.

Antenatal preparation

Nipple soreness is not related to the mother's colouring, nor to the toughness of her skin.

There is no evidence to support the commonly held belief that fair-skinned women are more likely to experience nipple problems (12–14). The persistence of this myth may result in unjustifiable numbers of fair/red/ auburn-haired women being dissuaded from breastfeeding; and problems, should they occur in such women, being regarded as unavoidable.

Nipple shape

Although antenatal examination of the nipples may have some predictive value, many women with poorly protractile nipples will be able to breastfeed successfully without treatment (15). They will probably need particular help with attaching their baby to the breast during the first feeds. There is as yet no evidence about the use of Woolwich shells in pregnancy for women with inverted or poorly protractile nipples. A multicentre trial on this subject is currently underway in the UK.

As the nipple plays little active part in the mechanism of milk release (see p. 5) breastfeeding success is likely to have more to do with good positioning than with nipple shape.

Nipple preparation

Although there are many variations in the recommended practices, they all fall into three major categories: some form of nipple friction, application of various creams or antenatal expression of colostrum. These practices have been evaluated by a number of researchers (12, 16, 17, 18), and no evidence has been found to support any of them.

The arguments on which they are based have been further undermined by studies which have found no differences between the incidence of nipple problems between multiparae and primiparae (19–21), which would be expected if nipple 'toughening' were effective.

Expression of colostrum

There is no justification for advising pregnant women to express colostrum regularly, on the grounds that it will improve subsequent lactation. Not only does it have no effect on milk flow or milk production (1, 22, 23) but it may dispose women to mastitis if the breast is traumatised (22). On the other hand there is no reason why a woman who wishes to satisfy her curiosity as to the nature of colostrum should be dissuaded from doing so (gently).

A pregnant woman who intends to breastfeed should be advised that no physical preparation of her breasts can ensure trouble-free feeding. Instead she should be taught the principles of good breastfeeding technique, and to regard any pain she may experience not as inevitable, but as a signal that she needs to improve her technique.

Postnatal care of the breasts
Cleanliness

Washing the breasts before each feed is no longer recommended, and mothers should be advised that adequate personal hygiene is all that is necessary. The use of soap, and the use of alcohol have both been shown to increase the incidence of nipple soreness (24). Sprays containing alcohol and chlorhexidine are ineffective in preventing nipple trauma (25, 26).

Creams and ointments

Of those that have been tested in controlled trials, stilboestrol cream and vitamin A and D concentrate (cod-

57

liver oil) have been shown to *increase* the incidence of nipple damage (13, 24); and lanolin, vitamin A and D ointment, vitamin B ointment (both in lanolin and petroleum base) and water repellent silicone barrier cream have been shown to be *ineffective* in preventing nipple damage (13, 24, 27). Tincture of benzoin, although not formally tested, contains 75–80% alcohol and might therefore be expected to increase the incidence of nipple damage. It is likely that any cream will alter the skin ecology in some way (28), and its use must always be justified.

Since there seems to be little evidence that any of the creams, ointments, sprays or tinctures frequently advocated is of any value in preventing nipple soreness, attention should be paid to ensuring that the baby is correctly positioned whenever he breastfeeds.

Limiting sucking time

This practice, which was first advocated in the early 1900s, was also a product of the mistaken belief that nipples needed toughening to promote pain-free feeding. Recent studies have shown that nipple soreness is not affected by the duration of the feed, but that limiting sucking time is likely to have an adverse effect on breastfeeding as a whole (29, 30).

Treatment of sore nipples

Most methods of treatment currently advocated (31) fall into two groups: (i) those that aim to heal the nipple by putting something on it (the 'magic wand' treatments), and (ii) those that aim to allow the nipple to heal spontaneously by removing or reducing the cause of the damage. No randomised controlled trial (RCT) has yet been done to assess the usefulness of any of the creams, sprays, lotions or ointments that, according to a recent study (31), are often recommended by midwives as treatments for sore nipples; there is thus no scientific basis for their use. Nor is there any scientific evidence to support the use of expressed breast milk or colostrum on the nipples after feeding (32).

Only one RCT has yet been conducted to assess the effectiveness of methods designed to remove or reduce damage (19) and this compared three methods: (i) taking the baby off the breast and expressing the milk, (ii) the use of a nipple shield, and (iii) repositioning the baby at the breast (although precisely what was understood by this term was not clearly defined).

Over the 48-hour period of the trial all methods were equally acceptable in producing nipple healing, but the use of the nipple shield proved to be highly unacceptable to mothers. Additionally, the use of a traditional nipple shield has also been shown (33) to reduce significantly the amount of milk available to the baby.

Resting and expressing
Repositioning

The two methods that did seem acceptable to the majority of mothers allocated to each one – 'repositioning' and 'resting and expressing' – were equally effective in producing nipple healing over the 48 hours of the trial Thus with both treatments the nipple had ceased to be traumatised.

However, the long term objective of treating sore nipples is to facilitate pain-free, successful breastfeeding. Logically, removing the baby from the breast will heal sore nipples, but only in the same way that not breastfeeding at all will 'prevent' them. Furthermore, removing the baby from the breast in order to heal nipples immediately creates the problem of maintaining milk production. A breast pump applies negative pressure to the end of the nipple, but it does not directly stimulate the nerve endings in the areola (34). Thus the prolactin surge that normally follows suckling (and is responsible, in part, for milk synthesis) is reduced or absent when a breast pump is used (35).

The other components in the maintenance of lactation are the effective removal of milk in response to the milking action provided by the baby's tongue and jaw (absent if a pump is used) and the active expulsion of milk in response to oxytocin release, the 'let down' reflex.

Less milk will be obtained from the breast in response to periodic expression compared with direct suckling (36). (This deficit was reduced by giving nasal oxytocin to mothers who needed to use a breast pump for any length of time (37).) On both counts therefore milk production begins to decline. (The use of a breast pump should not be

59

assumed to be a totally atraumatic process; in the trial referred to above (19), four of the six women with new nipple cracks at the end of 48 hours had been using a breast pump.)

Thus in terms of achieving the long term goal of pain-free, successful lactation, paying close attention to feeding technique ('repositioning') is likely to be far more effective than removing the baby from the breast ('resting and expressing').

Nipple shields

Nipple shields should not be used as a substitute for teaching the mother how to correct the problem of sore nipples by improving her feeding technique. Their use in the early days of lactation may lead to a conditioned rejection of the breast by the baby, which can be extremely difficult to correct. Prolonged use may also adversely affect the mother's milk supply, as less milk is made available to the baby as a result of less efficient milking action of the baby's tongue and jaw through the layer of rubber. This is particularly true of the traditional thick rubber nipple shields (33). (As yet there is no evidence on which to base statements about the effectiveness of silicone shields.)

Some mothers may benefit from the judicious use of a thin, latex rubber shield, principally if their nipples have been severely traumatised by incorrect positioning, and they choose not to 'rest and express'. They should bear in mind that milk transfer may be impaired (33) and compensate for this by offering the breast for longer.

Prevention and treatment of engorgement

This term needs defining as different people mean different things by it.

Vascular engorgement

Because lactation is anticipated, the body prepares the breast anatomically and physiologically (38). During the course of pregnancy, ductal and alveolar growth is stimulated (and milk secretion inhibited) by the high levels of placental oestrogen in the mother's bloodstream. When, after placental delivery, this has fallen to a point where it can no longer inhibit the action of prolactin, synthesis and secretion of milk can begin. This requires extensive cardiovascular changes in the mother, and blood flow to the breasts (and gastrointestinal tract and liver) is increased (39). The discomfort that the mother experiences in the first 2 4 days after birth will depend on the extent of the increase. The early changes are not due to the breasts being overfull with milk (40) and neither expression nor oxytocin administration are of value.

Milk engorgement

Since the initiation of the vascular changes in the breasts and the secretion of milk are both the result of the uninhibited action of prolactin, there is a degree of overlap between vascular engorgement and milk production. The milk, once secreted, is stored in the alveoli, which are surrounded by myoepithelial cells (see pp. 1–2). When the baby is correctly attached to the breast the oxytocin released by suckling causes these cells to contract and propel the milk forward into the lactiferous sinuses beneath the areola, where it can be removed by the baby. If the milk is not removed as it is formed – as regulated by the baby's need to go to the breast – either because the baby's access to the breast is restricted, or because of incorrect positioning once there, it is quite likely that as milk production rapidly increases the volume of milk in the breast will exceed the capacity of the alveoli to store it comfortably.

The subsequent over-distension of the alveoli causes the milk secreting cells to become flattened, drawn out and even to rupture (41), and further milk production begins to be suppressed. In some instances the pressure in the alveoli may be sufficiently high to force substances from the milk into the capillaries or connective tissues. This in turn will activate the mother's immune system – her pulse and temperature will rise, a red, painful area appears on the breast and the aching, flu-like feeling she experiences may be accompanied by rigors (42). These are the classic symptoms of non-infective mastitis which, if untreated, may progress to infective mastitis and even abscess formation (see below).

Prevention

Milk engorgement is almost always iatrogenic – it rarely

6

occurs when mothers are able to feed their babies 'on demand' day and night (43–45) (see pp. 30–31). It may be further prevented by ensuring that the baby is correctly attached on each occasion so that the milk is efficiently removed and the 'let-down' reflex effectively stimulated.

Treatment

If a breastfeeding woman develops milk engorgement, attention must first be paid to the possible cause. If the mother is attempting to regulate either the frequency or duration of the feeds she should be dissuaded from doing so. She may mistakenly believe that the baby must feed from both breasts at each feed (see p. 23). Her feeding technique should be observed and help given if necessary to ensure effective attachment. Sometimes gentle expressing to soften the breast prior to feeding is all that is necessary. Some women find this easier to do in a warm shower or bath. In most instances this should be sufficient. Only if the engorgement has progressed to the point of inflammation may it be necessary to express milk gently after the feed (by hand or by pump) until the engorgement has subsided (46). Cold compresses between feeds may also be comforting, although there is no evidence that this is generally effective.

Prevention and treatment of mastitis

The term 'mastitis' should not be regarded as synonymous with 'breast infection'. Although inflammation of the breast may be the result of an infective process, in 50% of cases it is not (46–48). Thus automatic recourse to antibiotic therapy may be inappropriate.

Non-infective mastitis

If the milk is not removed from the breast at the rate at which it is produced, the pressure in the alveoli will start to rise. This rise may be generalised, as in the case of engorgement, or localised, as a result of some specific internal or external obstruction, e.g. blocked duct bruising from trauma or rough handling, compression from fingers holding the breast, a tight brassiere or incorrect positioning. (A localised obstruction may sometimes be felt as a lump in the breast.) If this situation is not relieved the pressure in the alveoli may become sufficiently high to

62

cause milk substances to be forced out into the
surrounding tissue (see p. 61).

Infective mastitis

Breast infections may occur in the outer skin of the breast,
or within the glandular or connective tissue deeper in the
breast. Unless this is treated quickly, abscess formation
may take place.

Prevention of non-infective mastitis

This condition is often a consequence of engorgement, and
should be prevented in the same way. Localised
obstructions should be avoided by advising the woman not
to wear clothing that puts pressure on her breasts, to
handle her breasts gently to avoid bruising, not to grip her
breast tightly when supporting it while feeding and to treat
any lumpiness in the breast promptly by encouraging
drainage from that area, by improving positioning and
gently stroking the affected area downward towards the
nipple.

Correct positioning is also an essential part of the
prevention of this condition.

Prevention of infective mastitis

The epithelium of the breast and nipple may be damaged
by incorrect positioning of the baby at the breast, or
occasionally by the use of creams, lotions or sprays to
which the mother is sensitive and which subsequently
damage the skin (25).

Bacterial infection requires that organisms breach the
protective barrier of the skin, and are able to multiply in
spite of the body's defence system.

Once the skin is damaged, rapid multiplication of the
bacteria is encouraged by the prolonged use of breast
shells or nursing pads which keep the nipple wet. Other
factors include poor physical health, especially iron
deficiency which affects antibody production (45), poor
nutrition (49), the use of creams, lotions or sprays which
alter the skin's natural defences (25) and possibly
smoking, which may alter immune responses (50).
Unresolved non-infective mastitis may progress to
infective mastitis (46).

63

Treatment of mastitis

In the past any inflammation of the breast was likely to be treated with systemic antibiotics. This seems to be because it was not recognised that the inflammation was not necessarily caused by an infection (47, 48), and partly because then, as now, culturing milk samples took too long for the results to be used as the basis for starting treatment.

However, one study (46) suggests that an effective differential diagnosis can be made on the basis of a leucocyte and bacterial count of samples of breastmilk – a test that can be completed rapidly in a laboratory. The study found that women who were displaying the signs and symptoms of 'mastitis' but whose milk contained less than 10^6 leucocytes and less than 10^3 bacteria per ml needed no treatment other than to continue breastfeeding. Those with less than 10^6 leucocytes but more than 10^3 bacteria benefited from expressing milk after a feed as well as continuing to breastfeed. Only those with a leucocyte count in excess of 10^6 and a bacterial count in excess of 10^3 were deemed to be suffering from infective mastitis and required antibiotics in addition to breastfeeding and expressing after feeds.

Most antimicrobial drugs taken by the mother do not, in general, appear in her breastmilk in amounts sufficient to affect her nursing infant (51), although some adverse effects have been noted, principally rashes, diarrhoea and thrush (52). (These drugs may also produce similar side effects in the mother.) Thus it would be of benefit if, by employing some means of rapid, differential diagnosis, such as a modification of that described above, the infant of a mother who developed a breast inflammation was not, in consequence, automatically exposed to the possibility of such side effects.

In the absence of this facility, provided it was possible to monitor the mother closely, it might be appropriate to delay antibiotic therapy for 6–8 hours, whilst taking the corrective measures described above. If, however, there was no improvement during this time, a broad spectrum antibiotic (such as flucloxacillin) would be necessary.

If it is not possible to provide close professional supervision and support for a mother with mastitis, prophylactic antibiotics will be needed from the outset.

Finally, there is no justification for advising a lactating woman with mastitis to stop breastfeeding – indeed abrupt weaning appears to increase the chances that the woman will develop a breast abscess (48) (see also p. 72).

References

Influencing the decision to breastfeed

1. Beske EJ, Garvis MS 1982 Important Factors in Breastfeeding Success. Maternal and Child Nursing 7: 174–179
2. Ladas AK 1970 The Relationship of Information and Support to Behaviour, The La Leche League and Breastfeeding PHD Dissertation. Columbia University, New York
3. Kaplowitz DD 1983 The Effect of an Education Programme on the Decision to Breastfeed. Journal of Nutrition Education 15: 61–65
4. Switzky LT, Vietze P, Switzky HN 1979 Attitudinal and Demographic Predictors of Breastfeeding and Bottlefeeding Behaviour by Mothers of Six-Week-Old Infants. Psychological Reports 45: 3–14
5. Svejcar J 1977 Methodological Approaches to the Promotion and Maintenance of Breastfeeding. Klinische Paediatrie 189: 333–336
6. Kirk TR 1979 An Evaluation of the Impact of Breastfeeding Promotions in Edinburgh. Proceedings Nutrition Society 38: 77A
7. Gueri M, Jutsum P, White A 1979 Evaluation of a Breastfeeding Campaign in Trinidad. Bolatin Oficina Sanitoria Panamericana 86 (3): 189–195
8. Wiles LS 1984 The Effect of Prenatal Breastfeeding Education on Breastfeeding Success and Maternal Perception of the Infant. Journal of Obstetric, Gynaecologic and Neonatal Nursing 13: 253–257

Sustaining the decision to breastfeed

9. Johnson CA, Garza C, Nichols B 1984 A Teaching Intervention to Improve Breastfeeding Success. Journal of Nutrition Education 16: 19–22
10. Houston MJ 1985. In: Minchin MK Breastfeeding Matters. Alma Publications, Allen & Unwin, Australia pp 105–106
11. Sjolin S, Hofvander Y, Hillervick C 1979 A Prospective Study of Individual Courses of Breastfeeding. Acta Paediatrica Scandinavica 68: 521–529

Prevention of feeding problems

12. Scott-Brown MS, Hurlock JT 1975 Preparation of the Breast for Breastfeeding. Nursing Research. 24: 448–451
13. Gans B 1958 Breast and Nipple Pain in the Early Stages of Lactation. British Medical Journal October 4th: 830–834
14. Brockway L 1986 Hair Colour and Problems in Breastfeeding. Midwives Chronicle and Nursing Notes March: 66–67
15. Hytten FE 1954 Clinical and Chemical Studies in Lactation. IX. Breastfeeding in Hospital. British Medical Journal December 18th: 1447–1452

65

16. L'Esperance CM 1980 Pain or Pleasure: The Dilemma of Early Breastfeeding. Birth and the Family Journal 7(1): 21–26
17. Whitley N 1978 Preparation of the Breasts for Breastfeeding. A One Year Follow-up of 34 Mothers. Journal of Obstetric, Gynaecologic and Neonatal Nursing 7(3): 44–48
18. Clark M 1985 A Study of 4 Methods of Nipple Care Offered to Post Partum Mothers. New Zealand Nursing Journal 78: 16–18
19. Nicholson W 1985 Cracked Nipples in Breastfeeding Mothers – A Randomised Trial of Three Methods of Management. Newsletter of the Nursing Mothers of Australia 21(4): 7–10
20. Jones D 1984 Breastfeeding Problems. Nursing Times August 15th: 53–54
21. Gunther M 1945 Sore Nipples – Cause and Prevention. Lancet ii: 590–593
22. Ingelman-Sundberg A 1958 The Value of Antenatal Massage of the Nipples and Expression of Colostrum. Journal of Obstetrics and Gynaecology of the British Empire 65(3): 448–449
23. Waller H, Aschaffenburg R, Grant MW 1941 Biochemical Journal 35: 272

Postnatal care of the breasts

24. Newton N 1952 Nipple Pain and Nipple Damage. Journal of Pediatrics 41: 411–423
25. Slaven D, Harvey D, Craft I. A Double-blind Controlled Trial of Chlorhexidine in Aerosol Spray for the Prevention of Sore Nipples (unpublished). In: Inch S 1987 Difficulties in Breastfeeding – Midwives in Disarray? Journal of the Royal Society of Medicine 80: 53–57
26. Herd B, Feeney JG 1986 Two Aerosol Sprays in Nipple Trauma. The Practitioner 230: 31–38. *See also:* Inch S, Fisher C 1987 Antiseptic Sprays and Nipple Trauma. The Practitioner 230: 1037–1038
27. Shurtz AR et al 1978 Comparison of Nipple Care in the Puerperium with Powder and Ointment. Gerburtshilfe Frauenheik 38: 573–576
28. Minchin M 1985 Breastfeeding Matters. Alma Publications, Allen & Unwin, Australia, ch 4
29. Slaven S, Harvey D 1981 Unlimited Sucking Time Improves Breastfeeding. Lancet i: 392–393
30. Carvahlo M, Robertson S, Klaus M 1984 Does the Duration and Frequency of Early Breastfeeding Affect Nipple Pain? Birth 11(2): 81–84

Treatment of sore nipples

31. Garcia J, Garforth S 1985 A National Study of Policy and Practice in Midwifery. Available from: The National Perinatal Epidemilogy Unit, Radcliffe Infirmary, Oxford OX2 6HE
32. Hewat RJ, Ellis DJ 1987 A Comparison of the Effectiveness of Two Methods of Nipple Care. Birth 41: March 1, pp. 41–45
33. Woolridge MW, Baum D, Drewett RF 1980 Effect of a Traditional and of a New Nipple Shield on Sucking Patterns and Milk Flow. Early Human Development 4(4): 357–364

Successful breastfeeding

34. Howie PW 1985 Breastfeeding – A New Understanding. Midwives Chronicle and Nursing Notes July: 184–192
35. Howie PW, McNeilly AS, McArdle T, Smart L, Houston MJ 1980 The Relationship Between Suckling Induced Prolactin Response and Lactogenesis. Journal of Clinical Endocrinology and Metabolism 50: 670–673
36. Freidman EA, Sachtleben MR 1961 Oxytocin in Lactation. American Journal of Obstetrics and Gynecology 82: 846–855
37. Ruis H 1981 Oxytocin Enhances the Onset of Lactation Amongst Mothers Delivering Prematurely. British Medical Journal 283: 340–342

Prevention and treatment of engorgement

38. Smith VR 1974 The Mammary Gland – Development and Maintenance. Lactation. Academic Press, New York Vol 1
39. Lawrence R 1980 Breastfeeding – A Guide for the Medical Profession. CV Mosby, St. Louis
40. Ingelman-Sundberg A 1953 Early Puerperal Engorgement. Acta Paediatrica Scandinavica 32: 399–402
41. Dawson EK 1935 Edinburgh Medical Journal 42: 569
42. Gunther M 1973 Infant Feeding, Penguin
43. Fildes V 1979 Putting Mum in the Picture. Nursing Mirror 149(3): 22–24
44. Applebaum RM 1977 The Modern Management of Successful Breastfeeding. Pediatric Clinics of North America 241(1): 37–47
45. Minchin M 1985 Breastfeeding Matters. Allen & Unwin, Australia, p 163
46. Thomsen AC et al 1984 Course and Treatment of Milk Stasis, Non-infectious Inflammation of the Breast and Infectious Mastitis in Nursing Women. American Journal of Obstetrics and Gynecology 149(5): 492–495

Prevention and treatment of mastitis

47. Neibyl JR et al 1978 Sporadic (Non Epidemic) Puerperal Mastitis. Journal of Reproductive Medicine 20(2): 97–100
48. Marshall BR et al 1975 Sporadic Puerperal Mastitis. Journal of the American Medical Association 233(13): 1377–1379
49. Miranda R et al 1983 Effects of Maternal Nutritional Status on Immunological Substances in Human Colostrum and Milk. American Journal of Clinical Nutrition 37: 632–640
50. Kjellman NI 1981 Effects of Prenatal Smoking on IgE Levels in Children. Lancet i: 993
51. White GJ, White M 1984 Breastfeeding and Drugs in Human Milk. Veterinary and Human Toxicology vol 26 (suppl 1) p 3
52. Brodie MJ 1986 Drugs and Breastfeeding. The Practitioner 230: 483–485

Antenatal and postnatal considerations

Notes on less common problems

Baby vomiting blood   69
Blood in milk/colostrum   69
Blanching of the nipple (white nipple)   69
Thrush infection of the nipple   70
Contact dermatitis   70
Diabetes   70
Epilepsy   70
Anticoagulant therapy   70
Other drugs and breastfeeding   70
Mammary surgery   71
Cleft lip   71
Cleft palate   71
Down's syndrome   72
Tandem feeding   72
Breast abscess   72
Inverted nipples   72
AIDS and breastfeeding   73
Herpes simplex infection   74

Baby vomiting blood

Blood in vomited breast milk or in stools (melaena spuria) often originates from a damaged nipple. Breastfeeding should continue and the cause of the damage should be corrected (see pp. 58–60). If the diagnosis is uncertain, blood can be tested for adult or fetal haemoglobin.

Blood in milk/colostrum

This condition occurs infrequently and appears to be harmless. The cause is unclear and it usually resolves spontaneously as lactation is established; breastfeeding can continue. However, if the condition persists or the mother is anxious, it would seem prudent to seek informed medical opinion.

Blanching of the nipple (white nipple)

This painful condition may be associated with circulatory problems. Positioning of the baby should be checked as trauma may trigger a response. Helpful reported remedies include feeding in a warmer room, and drinking tea (which contains the vasodilator theophylline) before the feed.

69

Thrush infection of the nipple

Onset may follow a period of trouble-free feeding. The nipple and the areola are inflamed and painful during and between feeds. There may also be pain radiating through the breast after feeding. The baby may have obvious oral or anal thrush. Mother and baby should be thoroughly treated with an antifungicidal preparation. The mother is more likely to tolerate the discomfort when she knows there is a cure.

Contact dermatitis

Women may develop dermatitis of the nipple and breast from lanolin or other ointments, from chlorhexidine spray or from detergents in brassieres. All local applications should be stopped. If it is likely that the dermatitis is caused by the brassiere, the mother should use breast pads which are not plastic backed and wash her clothing in soap.

Diabetes

This is not a contraindication to breastfeeding. If the mother is insulin dependent her regime will be adjusted as part of her routine treatment. Her intention to breastfeed must be conveyed to her physician as she may require less insulin (1, 2).

Epilepsy

Drugs which are considered safe for pregnancy will be safe for breastfeeding, as they are more likely to pass the placental barrier than to be excreted in milk. If the mother is prone to seizures she should feed where the baby will come to no harm. (The breastfed baby is certainly at no greater risk than the bottle-fed one in such situations; and since a breastfeeding mother can lie down to feed, her baby may be at less risk.)

Anticoagulant therapy

Heparin and warfarin may safely be given while breastfeeding (3). Expert advice should be sought for other drugs.

Other drugs and breastfeeding

70

Most health authorities and health boards have a drug

information centre which will help with any enquiries about maternal medication during lactation. Otherwise, hospital pharmacies should be able to obtain the necessary information. In the case of commonly used drugs it is unlikely that the risks to the baby outweigh the benefits of breastfeeding. In almost all cases, a safer alternative drug can be found, or at worst breastfeeding need only be interrupted briefly (4).

Mammary surgery

Women can breastfeed successfully following unilateral mastectomy, provided that the other breast is functionally normal. Women who have had silicone implants or reduction mammoplasty may be able to breastfeed successfully as it is probable that both the nerve supply to the nipple and the ductal system necessary for sustained lactation will have been left intact in these cases. If the nipple has been resited it is most unlikely that breastfeeding will be possible.

Cleft lip

This should not cause any breastfeeding problems. Some surgeons encourage breastfeeding soon after plastic surgery; others advise an initial period of spoon-feeding.

Cleft palate

This defect, unless it is very small, causes major problems. The baby cannot create a seal between his mouth and the breast and cannot therefore make a teat out of the breast and nipple, which is the prerequisite of efficient milk removal. The defect can be 'closed' with a feeding plate or palate seal, but even with this most babies still have great difficulty breastfeeding. It appears that the sucking reflex is most effectively stimulated by the sensation of the nipple against the baby's palate (5, 6) and the stimulus is thus greatly reduced with this condition. Mothers who want to feed their babies with their own milk can do so by expressing their breastmilk and feeding it to the baby using a special bottle, teat or spoon. Breastfeeding can be attempted, and may even be successful if the mother has a large, elastic breast and a ready milk ejection reflex, but it is usually necessary to supplement while breastfeeding with a nursing supplementer (7).

71

Down's syndrome

These babies need extra help during the initiation period, and much time and patience is required to ensure that they are properly attached to the breast at each feed. The mother may need to express her milk while this learning process is proceeding. The benefits of breastfeeding assume particular importance for these babies.

Tandem feeding

Midwives may occasionally encounter a mother who continues to breastfeed throughout her subsequent pregnancy, and breastfeeds both the newborn baby and his sibling afterwards. There is no evidence to suggest that this is harmful for the mother or her children. It is important, however, that the newborn baby's needs are met first. (In practice many young children cease feeding during the mother's pregnancy. It is suggested that the volume reduces and the taste changes.) Nipple soreness is commonly reported by mothers who breastfeed through pregnancy.

Breast abscess

Abscess formation requires that organisms breach the protective barrier of the skin and multiply in spite of the body's defence system. Abscesses may form superficially, often near the areola, or deep within the substance of the breast. These deeper abscesses are often the result of unresolved non-infective mastitis which has damaged the tissues and made them vulnerable to infection. Once an abscess has formed, it may be necessary to incise the breast in order to drain it. Unless the position of the incision makes it impossible, breastfeeding should continue as this is likely to speed healing (8). Alternatively, the abscess may be aspirated, which avoids the necessity for hospital admission (9). Feeding should continue uninterrupted on the unaffected side and the baby returned to the affected side as quickly as possible.

Inverted nipples

Although uncommon, inverted nipples present a real challenge to midwives. There is to date no evidence that either Woolwich shells or the use of the Hoffman technique are beneficial. Nipple shape (or lack of nipple)

72

is less important than the protractility of the surrounding tissue, as it is this which determines the baby's ability to make an effective 'teat' from the breast (5).

No prediction of the ultimate success of breastfeeding should be made on the basis of antenatal inspection of a woman's nipples, as dramatic changes in shape often take place around parturition (see p. 6). If the midwife is initially unable to attach the baby to the breast effectively, lactation can be initiated and sustained with a breast pump, and further attempts made when the milk is 'in' and the breasts have softened.

Skilled help with positioning the baby in the first few days is particularly helpful in these cases.

AIDS and breastfeeding

Guidance concerning breastfeeding by women at risk of HIV infection and amplification of the guidance on human milk banking is contained in a Department of Health letter 'HIV Infection, Breastfeeding and Human Milk Banking in the United Kingdom' (PL/CMO(89)4; PL/CNO(89)3). Women who are HIV antibody positive should be advised that it is prudent to avoid breastfeeding. Women who are at risk of HIV infection and are HIV negative or decline serotesting should receive counselling. Some may need to be advised about the risks of transmission as if they were HIV positive. Serotesting should be made available.

Herpes simplex infection

If a mother has a lesion on her breast, it should be regarded as infectious for the first 5 days (10). During this time the baby may be at risk of infection if fed directly from the breast. If this is thought to be the case, milk should be expressed (to maintain lactation) and the expressed milk fed to the baby after a few hours have elapsed, using a spoon or bottle. (Since the mother will have been infectious before the lesion developed, her milk will contain antibodies to the virus. These will remain in the milk after expression and afford some measure of protection for the baby. Allowing a few hours to elapse between expressing the milk and giving it to the baby may mean a lowered level of the virus in the milk as a result of its antiviral properties (11).)

73

7

If the lesion is not on the breast, and the baby is not likely to come into direct contact with it, breastfeeding can continue, but the mother should be advised to pay particular attention to washing her hands before feeding her baby (12).

References

1. Whichelow MJ, Doddridge MC 1983 Lactation in Diabetic Women. British Medical Journal 287: 649
2. Miller DL 1977 Birth and Long Term Unsupplemented Breastfeeding in 17 Insulin Dependent Mothers. Birth and the Family Journal 4: 65–70
3. L'E Orme M et al 1977 May Mothers Given Warfarin Breastfeed Their Infants? British Medical Journal June 18th pp 1564–1565
4. Wilson JT 1981 Drugs in Breastmilk. Lancaster MTP
5. Gunther M 1955 Instinct and the Nursing Couple. Lancet i: 575–578
6. Peiper A 1963 Cerebral Function in Infancy and Childhood. 3rd edn. Consultants Bureau, New York, pp 418–420
7. Danner SC 1986 Breastfeeding Your Cleft Lip/Palate Baby. Lactation Consultant Series, Avery Press, New Jersey or pamphlet available from: Birth and Life Bookstore, PO Box 70625, Seattle, WA 98107, USA
8. Benson EA, Goodman MA 1970 An Evaluation of the Use of Stilboestrol and Antibiotics in the Early Management of Acute Puerperal Breast Abscess. British Journal of Surgery 57: 258
9. Dixon JM 1988 Repeated Aspiration of Breast Abscess in Lactating Women. British Medical Journal December 10th pp 1517–1518
10. Spruance SL, Overall JC, Kern ER, Krueger GG, Pham V, Miller W 1977 The Natural History of Recurrent Herpes Simplex Labialis. New England Journal of Medicine 297(2): 57–70
11. Cerutti E, White G 1981 Management of Mother Infant Problems During Lactation. Taped at the LLL Physicians' Seminar 1981. Available from LLL, for address see Appendix 1.
12. Yeager AS, Ashley RL, Corey L 1983 Transmission of Herpes Simplex Virus from Father to Neonate. Journal of Paediatrics 103(6): 905–907

Breastfeeding under special circumstances

Preterm infants   75
Caesarean section   //
Twins   77
Triplets   77
Establishing lactation with an electric pump   77
Babies being cared for in units other than maternity units   78

One of the midwife's main roles is to ensure that women who wish to lactate and breastfeed do so successfully. In circumstances where the mother is under additional pressure or the normal mechanisms for ensuring successful lactation are interrupted, the mother will need particular help.

In neonatal intensive and special care units, for example, the nursing priority may be to ensure that the baby makes rapid progress and is speedily discharged.

Sometimes, these objectives, with their emphasis on tube feeding and/or preterm formula, may be at odds with establishment of the mother's lactation. Once the child is returned to his mother's care, it is she who will be solely responsible for his nutrition, and it would be regrettable if the opportunity for long term breastfeeding was sacrificed at an early stage in favour of short term gains. Midwives should do all they can to protect the mother's lactation in these circumstances.

Preterm infants

For mothers who have successfully initiated lactation with an electric pump, the transition from tube feeds to breastfeeding can be very difficult. The preterm tube-fed baby is deprived of the sucking and swallowing experiences he has had in utero, and so may be artificially delayed in his competence at feeding. If he has received his mother's milk by bottle he may need help adapting his feeding technique, and his mother will need particularly caring support at this time.

Babies are naturally equipped for feeding at the breast, so once they are developmentally competent they should not be denied the opportunity to feed on the grounds that

75

it would be 'too long'. It has been demonstrated (1) that preterm infants who are able to suck find breastfeeding less 'demanding' than bottle-feeding.

Recent studies have also shown that preterm infants allowed intermittent sucking on a 'blind teat' gained weight more rapidly than those who were not. It is possible that sucking facilitates the utilisation of tube-fed milk (2, 3). (This may be due to release of lingual lipase during sucking.) Allowing preterm infants to suckle at their mother's breast as soon as they are able would therefore be of benefit both to the baby and the mother.

Babies are neurologically and developmentally competent to suck and swallow at 32 weeks gestation, and experience at breastfeeding may aid maturation of the process. However, attempting to provide sucking experience with either a bottle teat or a dummy may be detrimental to some in the long term, as the techniques required for feeding from a breast and a bottle are quite different from each other (see pp. 13–14).

Babies as small as 1300–1400 g can successfully breastfeed (1), if hospital staff are well informed and hospital structures supportive. Excellent reviews of the problems of feeding low birth weight babies are available free of charge from the World Health Organization (4).

HIV and milk banking

Donor breast milk has a variety of important uses, ranging from the early feeds of the very small preterm (24–28 weeks) who seem to tolerate breast milk better than any other milk (5), to avoiding the use of cow's milk on the rare occasions when a breastfed baby is temporarily unable to take the breast.

Although concern about the possibility of the spread of the AIDS virus through the user of donor milk has resulted in the closure of many milk banks, recent research strongly suggests that pasteurisation eliminates any risk of the transmission of HIV (6).

Guidance issued by the Chief Medical Officer and endorsed by the Department of Health's Expert Advisory Group on AIDS recommends that women at risk of HIV infection should not donate milk intended for other women's babies.

Women willing to donate should be given an

explanatory leaflet about the reasons for self-exclusion by women at risk and the significance of the HIV test. An HIV antibody test must be performed and a negative result received before the donor's milk can be accepted (7).

Caesarean section

There is no evidence to support the long established belief that caesarean section itself has any deleterious effect on the establishment of lactation. The mother will probably require more help to find a comfortable feeding position and with attaching the baby to the breast in the first few days than she would if she had been vaginally delivered (8).

Twins

Nature is generous, and initially most women have a milk supply that is sufficient to feed two babies. Provided that both babies feed well there will continue to be enough for both. The mother should be encouraged to feed each baby individually during the early days so that the common early problems can be resolved efficiently. Each baby may have its own breast, or they may be switched at each feed. Some mothers will prefer to continue feeding the babies separately, some prefer to feed them simultaneously, and some will adapt according to the babies' natural feeding pattern (9) (see also Appendix 2).

Triplets

There are many recorded cases of triplets being successfully breastfed, but it requires a very committed mother and a lot of extra help and support (10).

Establishing lactation with an electric pump

There is little similarity between the action of a breast pump and the action of a baby feeding at the breast. It is also known that less prolactin is released when a breast pump is used than when the baby feeds directly (11). In spite of this, many women succeed in initiating lactation by using a breast pump. However, unless the baby is able to start feeding directly during the 2nd or 3rd week of life, the supply may begin to diminish, possibly as a result of falling prolactin levels (11). It is therefore of particular importance that further suppression does not occur as a

77

result of engorgement, and the mother be encouraged to express milk as frequently (and as efficiently) as possible (12). As with breastfeeding, no specific timing restrictions should be imposed on the length of each session, and the mother should be encouraged to continue as long as a reasonable volume can be obtained; she should avoid pressing the funnel too hard against the breast. It may also be helpful to support the breast from beneath. However, unlike breastfeeding, it may be beneficial to switch from side to side during the session.

Occasional breastfeeds should also be encouraged, if possible, as these will help to maintain the supply. The mother should be reassured that the pump is less efficient than a baby at milking the breast, and that she may well be capable of producing more milk than she can obtain by pumping.

In some circumstances, hand expression may be more appropriate or acceptable, and there is evidence to suggest that this technique results in higher prolactin levels (11).

There are also several designs of hand pump available which are quite adequate once lactation is established, but as they are more tiring to use and less efficient than expression by hand or by electric pump expression, initiating lactation with a hand pump may be more difficult than with the other two methods.

Midwives should be aware that breast pumps are a potential source of infection (13). Mothers should be given sterile tubing and 'safety' bottles on each occasion that they use the pump and should be carefully instructed in its use. Particular care must be taken to prevent milk entering the interior of the pump, and the collecting bottle must be clearly marked to indicate the maximum permissible volume. A record should be kept of all pump users and the pumps should be examined bacteriologically at regular intervals.

Babies being cared for in units other than maternity units

There may be special circumstances where babies are cared for in units without midwives being present, e.g., neonatal surgical units, paediatric wards). Midwives should consider how best to give support to those mothers who wish to breastfeed.

Successful breastfeeding

References

1. Berbaum J, Periera G, Peckham G 1982 Increased Oxygenation with Non-nutritive Sucking During Gavage Feeding in Premature Infants. Paediatric Research 16, 278A Abs 1199

2. Meier P, Cranston-Anderson J 1987 Responses of Small Preterm Infants to Bottle and Breast-Feeding. Maternal & Child Nursing 12: (March–April): 97–105

3. Field T, Ignatoff E, Tringer S et al 1982 Non-nutritive Sucking During Tube Feedings: Effects on Preterm Neonates in an Intensive Care Unit. Paediatrics 70: 381–384

4. World Health Organization; Distribution and Sales Service, 1211 Geneva 27, Switzerland or by mail order from: HMSO Publications Centre, 51 Nine Elms Lane, London SW8 5DR

5. Lucas A 1987 AIDS and Human Milk Bank Closures. Lancet i: pp 1092–3

6. Eglin RP, Wilkinson AR 1987 HIV Infection and Pasteurisation of Breastmilk. Lancet i: p 1093

7. HIV Infection, Breastfeeding and Human Milk Banking in the UK (PL/CMO(89)4; PL/CNO(89)3). Available from: Health Publications Unit, No 2 Site, Heywood, Lancashire OL10 2PZ

8. Lewis PJ, Devenish C, Kahn C 1980 Controlled Trial of Metachlorpramide in the Initiation of Breastfeeding. British Journal of Clinical Pharmacology 9: 217–219

9. Saint L, Maggiore P, Hartmann PE 1986 Yield and Nutrient Content of Milk in 8 Women Breastfeeding Twins and 1 Woman Breastfeeding Triplets. British Journal of Nutrition 56: 49–58

10. MacDonald D. More Than One. Ian Henry, Hornchurch, Essex

11. Howie PJ 1985 Breastfeeding – A New Understanding. Midwives Chronicle and Nursing Notes. July: 184–192

12. Howie PJ, McNeilly AS, McArdle T, Smart L, Houston MJ 1980 The Relationship Between Suckling-induced Prolactin Response and Lactogenesis. Journal of Clinical Endocrinology and Metabolism 50: 670–673

13. Moloney AC, Quoraishi AH, Parry P, Hall V 1987 A Bacteriological Examination of Breast Pumps. Journal of Hospital Infection 9: 169–174

Appendix 1
National and International
Voluntary Organisations

National Voluntary Organisations

In many areas, traditional family support systems no longer exist, so that mothers are isolated. Where extended families still exist, support may come at the price of inaccurate information about breastfeeding. Midwives can help mothers to find a network of friends by giving them the addresses of the following organisations:

National Childbirth Trust
Breastfeeding Promotion Group
Alexandra House, Oldham Terrace
Acton
London W3 6NH
Tel: 081–992 8637

Twins and Multiple Births Association
41 Fortuna Way
Grimsby,
South Humberside
DN 37 9SJ

La Leche League
Breastfeeding Help and Information
BM 3424
London WC1V 6XX
Tel: 071–242 1278

Baby Milk Action Coalition
6 Regent Terrace
Cambridge
CBZ 1AA
Tel: 0223–464420

Association of Breastfeeding Mothers
7 Maybourne Close, Springfield Road
London SE26 6HQ
Tel: 081–676 0965

These organisations also supply information in accordance with these guidelines, by phone (24 hours a day, 7 days a week) and in leaflets and books. Their free leaflets contain useful information, and also have local and national contact addresses on them.

Midwives can assist by handing these leaflets to women antenatally, who can then make friends among the community of local mothers, and inform themselves about common breastfeeding problems and how to overcome them.

Before they leave the ward, mothers may appreciate receiving leaflets or cards giving deatils about the support organisations.

International Voluntary Organisations

Internationally, breastfeeding support and action organisations can be located by writing to:

GIFA (Geneva Infant Feeding Association),
PO Box 157, 1211 Geneva 19, SWITZERLAND
(Publishes breastfeeding briefs, useful update service)

IBFAN Africa
PO Box 34308, Nairobi, KENYA

Action for Corporate Accountability,
3255 Hennepin Ave S. Minneapolis, MN55, USA
(Publishes IBFAN News)

LLLI (La Leche League International),
9615 Minneapolis Ave, Franklin Park, IL 60131, USA
(Free catalogue; publishes breastfeeding abstracts)

IOCU (International Organisation of Consumer Unions)
PO Box 1045, Penang, MALAYSIA

NMAA (Nursing Mothers' Association of Australia),
PO Box 231, Nunawading, Victoria, AUSTRALIA
(Free catalogue of useful materials)

Appendix 2
Further Reading

Chalmers I, Enkin M, Keirse NJC (eds) 1989 **Effective Care in Pregnancy and Childbirth.** Oxford University Press, chs. 21, 80, 81

Greasley V 1986 **Breastfeeding. In:** Nursing – The Add-on Journal of Clinical Nursing. 3rd series. Vol 3 (2): 63–70

La Leche International 1981 **The Art of Breastfeeding** (the anglicised version of 'The Womanly Art of Breastfeeding') USA. LLLl. Available from: La Leche League. See Appendix 1

Minchin M 1985 **Breastfeeding Matters,** Alma Publications, Allen and Unwin, Australia. Obtainable direct from: PO Box 39, Wendouree, Victoria 3355, Australia. Obtainable in the UK from: The National Childbirth Trust. See Appendix 1

Renfrew M, Fisher C, Arms S 1990 **Bestfeeding:** getting breastfeeding right for you. An illustrated guide. Celestial Arts Available from: Dept B Airlift Book Co, 26/28 Eden Grove, London N7 8EF

Stanway P, Stanway A 1983 **Breast is Best** 2nd edn. Pan Books, London

Index

A

Abscess, breast, 65, 72
Additional fluids, *see* Fluids
Addresses of national and
    international voluntary
    organisations, 81–2
Advice on first feeds, 25–7
Afterpains, 1
AIDS, *see* HIV infection
Allergic reactions to milk
    substitutes, 44, 46
Ampullae, 1
Antenatal classes, 54
Antenatal preparation of breast,
    53, 56–7
Antibiotics/antimicrobials for
    mastitis, 64
Anti-coagulant drugs, 70
Anti-epileptic drugs, 70
Appetite, infant, 10–11
Areola, amount visible, 18
Attachment of baby, correct, 4, 6
    indications, 18–19

B

Baby/infant
    appetite and intake variability/
        regulation, 10–11
    caesarean section-born, 77
    contact with mother, 55
    fluids for, *see* Fluids
    health and wellbeing,
        monitoring, 33–6
    in non-maternity units, 78
    positioning, *see* Positioning
    preterm, 75–6
    sleeping place, 31–3
    as source of encouragement to
        breastfeed, 55
    stripping of milk by, active, 2, 3
    sucking, *see* Sucking
    supporting, 18
    twins and triplets, 77
    vomiting of blood, 69
Banking, milk, 76–7
Bedding in, 31–3
Blanching of nipple, 69
Blood
    in milk/colostrum, 69

vomiting of, by baby, 69
Bottle feeding
    breastfeeding and, qualitative
        differences, 13–14
    milk tokens for, 47
Bowel movements, *see* Stools
Breast
    abscess, 65, 72
    antenatal preparation, 53, 56–7
    one or both offered, 28–9
    postnatal care, 57–8
    pregnancy and parturition-
        related changes, 6–7
    supporting and presenting,
        16–17, 17
Breast pump, 59, 60, 77–8
    lactation established with, 77–8
Breastfeed, decision to, 53–5
    influencing, 53–4
    sustaining, 54–5
Breastfeeding
    physiology, *see* Physiology of
        breastfeeding
    problems, 56–7, 58, 65, 69–74
        less common, 69–74
        prevention, 56–7, 62, 63
    in special circumstances, 75–9
    tandem, 72
Breastmilk, *see* Milk

C

Caesarean section, babies born by,
    77
Calories for mother, additional,
    45–6
Childbirth (parturition), breast
    changes during, 6–7
Classes, antenatal, 54
Cleanliness, breast, 57
Cleft lip and palate, 71
Code for Marketing of Breastmilk
    Substitutes, WHO, 47–9
Colostrum
    blood in, 69
    composition, explaining to
        mother, 27
    expression, 57
Complementary feeds, 41–4
Compression, waves/cycles of, 4,
    5

85

Contact, of baby with mother, 55
Contact dermatitis, 70
Contraceptive effect of
    breastfeeding, 30–1
Cot death, 32
Cow's milk, allergic reactions,
    44
Creams, 58

D

Death, cot, 32
Decision to breastfeed, *see*
    Breastfeed
Defaecation, *see* Stools
Dehydration, 41
Delivery room, first feed in, 26
Dermatitis, contact, 70
Diabetes, 70
Diet, maternal, modifications,
    45–9
Donor milk, 76–7
Down's syndrome, 72
Drugs and breastfeeding, 70–1
Duration of feeds, 9–10, 27–9
    unrestricted, 27–9

E

Electric pump, *see* Breast pump
Energy requirements of mother,
    additional, 45–6
Engorgement, 60–2
    milk, 61
    prevention, 62
    treatment, 62
    vascular, 60–1
Epilepsy, 70
Expressing, resting and, 59–60
Expression, colostrum, 57

F

Faeces, *see* Stools
Father encouraging breastfeeding,
    55
Feed(s), *see also* Breastfeed;
    Breastfeeding
    duration, *see* Duration
    first, 20–1, 25–7
        advice and support, 25–7
        suggestion for, 20–1
    frequency, *see* Frequency

mother's position/posture, 21–4
    night time, *see* Night
    supplementary/complementary,
        41–4
    unrestricted, 27–30
First feed, *see* Feed(s)
Fluids, additional
    for infant, 41–4
        hazards, 42–4
    for mother, 45
Free samples of breastmilk
        substitutes, provision, 47
Frequency of feeds, 10, 29–30
    unrestricted, 29–30

G

Growth pattern, weight
    measurement in
    determination of, 34–5

H

Hand, mother's use of left or right,
    16–17
Head position, baby's, 16
Health, baby's, monitoring, 33–6
Help (to/for mother), 14, 19–20,
    25–36
    direct, ways of giving, 19–20
    factors shown not to, 41–52
    factors shown to, 25–36
    when to offer, 14
Herpes simplex virus infection and
    breastfeeding, 73–4
HIV infection (and AIDS)
    breastfeeding and, 73
    milk banking and, 76–7
Hormones, lactational, 1–3
Hygiene, 57

I

Infant, *see* Baby/infant
Infections, 70, 71, 72
    breast pumps as source of, 78
    nipple, 70
Infective mastitis, 61, 63, 64–5
Intake by infant, variability and
    regulation of, 10–11
International voluntary
    organisations, 82
Inverted nipples, 72–3

Successful breastfeeding

J

Jaundice, 42
Jaw action, 18

L

Labour (parturition), breast
    changes during, 6–7
Lactation, *see* Milk
Let-down reflex, 2, 3, 59
Lip (baby's), 18
    cleft, 71
Lying down, feeding whilst, 21–2

M

Mammary surgery, 71
Mastitis, 61, 62–5
    infective, 61, 63, 64–5
        prevention, 63
    non-infective, 61, 62–3
        prevention, 63
    treatment, 64–5
Meconium, 35, 36
Milk, breast, *see also* Physiology
    banking (=donor milk), 76–7
    blood in, 69
    composition
        explaining to mother, 27
        non-uniformity, 3
    ejection/explusion reflex, 2, 3,
        59
    engorgement, 61
    production and secretion
        (lactation), 1–3
        establishment with electric
            pump, 77
        at night, 30
        over-, 28
    release, 3–6
    stripping/removal by baby of,
        active, 2, 3
    substitutes, 44, 47–9
        allergic reactions, 44, 46
        promotion/marketing, 47–9
Milk tokens for bottle feeding, 47
Monitoring of baby's health and
    wellbeing, 33–6
Mother (baby's)
    contact of baby with, 55
    dietary modifications, 45–9
    hand use, left or right, 16–17
    helping the, *see* Help

posture, 20–4
sleeping, 31, 33
teaching the, 54, 54–5
Mother (mother's) discouraging
    breastfeeding, 55
Multiple births, 77

N

National voluntary organisations,
    81–2
Neck position, baby's, 16
Night feeds, 30–3
    value, 30–1
Nipple(s)
    blanching (=white nipple), 69
    infections, 70
    inverted, 72–3
    preparation, 57
    problems (in general), 56
    shape, 56–7
        pregnancy and parturition-
            related changes in, 6–7
    soreness, 58–9, 69–70, 72–3
        prevention, 58
        treatment, 58–9
Nipple shields, 60
Nose, baby's, 16

O

Ointments, 58
Ovulation, prolactin levels
    suppressing, 30–1
Oxytocin release, 1–2

P

Pains
    after-, 1
    with milk ejection, 2
    as warning signal, 6
Palate, cleft, 71
Parturition, breast changes during,
    6–7
Physiology of breastfeeding/
    lactation, 1–7
    explaining to mother, 27
Pillows, supporting, 21, 23
Positioning
    of baby, 3–6, 13–24
        re-, 59–60
    of mother, 20–4

Postnatal considerations, 53–67
Posture, mother's, 20–4
Pregnancy
    breast changes during, 6–7
    colostrum expression in, 57
Preterm/premature infants, 75–6
Prolactin levels, 1
    night feeds and, 30–1
    ovulation suppression and, 30–1
Psychological components of
        successful breastfeeding,
        25, 26
Pump, breast, see Breast pump

R

Reflex
    let-down (ejection/expulsion), 2,
        3, 59
    rooting, 3
Resting and expressing, 59–60
Rooming in, 31
Rooting reflex, 3

S

Scissor grip, discouraging, 17
Seated, feeding whilst being, 21–2
Shields, nipple, 60
Sitting up, feeding whilst, 21–2
Sleeping
    by baby, location, 31
    by mother, 31, 33
Soreness, nipple, see Nipple
Soya based formula, allergic
        reactions, 44
Stools, 35–6
    very loose, 46
Substitutes, breastmilk, promotion/
        marketing, 47–9
Sucking by infant, 3–6
    in bottle feeding vs
        breastfeeding, 13

cycle, 5
    explaining to mother, 27
    time, limiting, 27–8, 58
Supplementary feeds, 41–4
Support (encouragement) with
        breastfeeding, 54–5
    at first feed, 25–7
Support (physical)
    of the baby, 18
    of the breast, 16–17, 17
    of the mother, 21, 23
Surgery, mammary, 71

T

Tandem feeding, 72
Teaching the mother, 54, 54–5
Thrush infection of nipple, 70
Tongue, baby's, 16
Triplets, 77
Twins, 77

V

Vascular engorgement, 60–1
Voluntary organisations, national
        and international, 81–2
Vomiting of blood by baby, 69

W

Weighing, test, 44–5
Weight, baby's
    gain, 34–5
    monitoring, 34–5
    variations, 35
Wellbeing, baby's, monitoring,
        33–6
White nipple, 69
WHO International Code for
        Marketing of Breastmilk
        Substitutes, 47–9

Successful breastfeeding